The Cancer Journey

Positive Steps To Help Yourself Heal

First published in Great Britain by Noble House,
63 Church Road, Hauxton, Cambridge, CB22 5HS

A CIP catalogue record of this book is available from the British Library

Trade paperback Isbn: 978-1-9075712-4-4
Ebook Isbn: 978-0-9570072-1-5

Edited by Jacqueline Burns, www.londonwritersclub.com

Text Design by Two Associates
Cover Design by Kate Sayer

Set in Gill Sans

Printed and bound by CPI Group (UK) Ltd, Croydon, CR0 4YY

2 4 6 8 10 9 7 5 3 1

The Cancer Journey

Positive Steps To Help Yourself Heal

Dr Pam Evans, Polly Noble and Nicholas Hull-Malham

The Cancer Journey

Acknowledgements

The idea for this book came from the brilliant mind of our fabulous mentor coach Suzy Greaves who, realising we were all planning to write books about our individual journeys, suggested we might consider collaborating. It was a fantastically inspired thought, and Suzy's enthusiasm and encouragement have been with us every step of the way, and for this we are truly grateful.

Our greatest debt is of course to our families and loved ones who, as well as giving of themselves unstintingly when we needed them during our treatments, have continued to be our greatest source of love, thoughtfulness and support throughout. We doubt they know just how much we love and appreciate them.

Katherine, thank you for offering to write the foreword for the book, your unflagging support of our work and for always being interested and keen to help in anyway. We are truly grateful to you.

To the many friends who have been there for us with words of encouragement, valuable feedback on the manuscript and enthusiastic championing for us to get the book published, we are especially grateful. Although we wrote the book and take full responsibility for its contents, in a sense it is not entirely our own. Throughout our journeys we have learned so much from the many friends we have met along the way, that we must also express our heartfelt thanks to them for sharing their experiences to help smooth our paths.

We also want to express our gratitude to John Welch whose support and encouragement to get the book into print has made it possible for all three of us to fulfil a dream.

Polly, Pam and Nick xxx

CONTENTS

CHAPTER 5
Taking Care of Your Emotional Needs

Part 2 – Listen To Your Body and Take Control

CHAPTER 6
Self-Help Techniques

CHAPTER 7
Pamper Your Body & Soul – Holistic/Complementary Therapies

CHAPTER 8
Express Yourself – Live Life, Be Brave, Find the New You!

CHAPTER 9

What Family and Friends Can Do To Help

Part 3- Living and Eating Consciously

CHAPTER 10

Eating Consciously

CHAPTER 11

Recipes – Release Your Inner Nigella or Jamie!

CHAPTER 12:
Potions and Lotions

Conclusion

Glossary

Resources

The Cancer Journey

10

Foreword

When my father was diagnosed with cancer in 1995, I was 15 years old. I had so many questions to ask but didn't want to upset my parents so kept them to myself. The only other person I knew who had had cancer was my best friend's mum and as she had passed away only 6 months previously, the last thing I thought she needed was to be explaining to me what was about to happen to my dad.

This book is exactly what I needed then. It's the go-to handbook for anyone with a diagnosis or for the loved ones of someone with cancer. It tells you the things your doctor won't, from what to wear on those dreaded chemo days and how to lessen the side effects, to how to boost your energy with superfoods, how to deal with the emotions of living with cancer as well as telling loved ones what NOT to say – allowing them to avoid embarrassing faux pas!

The advice in this book comes from Polly, Pam and Nick and is heartfelt, compassionate, thoughtful and above all, extremely useful. Polly has been a dear friend of mine for nearly 10 years. Her advice is always practical, precise, inspirational and comes from the heart. Having been through this themselves, they have been able to create a book which provides the reader with bite-sized chunks of the things you need to know to help you conquer the ups and downs of the cancer journey.

My life has been touched by cancer several times now. I know how important and vital this information is and I strongly believe it is a must have for anyone affected by cancer.

Katherine Jenkins

A proportion of the profits from this book will be donated to UK cancer charities including:

The Nicholas Hull-Malham Lymphoma Trust
    – Hammersmith Hospital
Marie Curie Cancer Care
Macmillan Cancer Support
Teenage Cancer Trust

About the Authors

Pam Evans

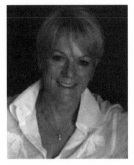

Pam worked in medical research for more than 25 years focusing largely on cancer therapies and adjuncts to cancer therapy and has a PhD in Medicine. While employed in the pharmaceutical/biotechnology industry she also trained as a career coach and has since expanded this knowledge and experience into the area of coaching those with life threatening illnesses. Following retirement from medical research, Pam retrained as a holistic therapist and works on a voluntary basis for Macmillan Cancer Support. She herself was diagnosed with breast cancer in 2006 and has fully recovered following a mastectomy. For more information about Pam's coaching business please visit **www.willtolivecoaching.com**

Polly Noble

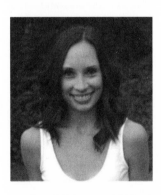

In 2005, aged 24, Polly was diagnosed with cervical cancer and treated with surgery, chemotherapy and radiotherapy. Since then, Polly has become passionate about health and nutrition and teaching others what they can do to empower themselves and take back the reins on their own health. She is a qualified Holistic Health Coach and helps others to create health and happiness in their lives.

As of February 2010, she is once again on the cancer train and is exploring a more natural method to healing her body using some of the techniques set out in this book. For more information you can visit **www.pollynoble.com** where she writes a personal blog and shares with others her knowledge and passion on health and healing.

Nicholas Hull-Malham

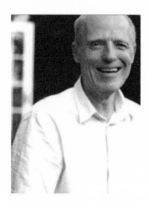

Nicholas worked in the entertainment industry before he trained in journalism at the London College of Print. He was a regular contributor to Disability Times newspaper for over four years and a deep interest in the human psyche led him to train as a psychotherapist and NLP Practitioner.

Two bouts of cancer made profound changes on Nick's life. One of those changes was becoming a stand up comic after his first cancer diagnosis. Nick also wrote a monthly self help column in GT magazine and is the creator of **www.laughingwithcancer.com**

Following his second diagnosis of cancer Nick also developed Parkinson's Disease but carried on living life to the full, passionate about making the most of every moment regardless of illness. Shortly after embarking on writing this book Nick was diagnosed with cancer for a third time but carried on seeing the manuscript almost completed. Following a stem-cell transplant Nicholas succumbed to pneumonia and sadly passed away.

The Cancer Journey
Positive Steps To Help Yourself Heal

Introduction

There's very little in this life which can turn our world upside down quite like the diagnosis of cancer. Our busy lives drop away and we become aware, as never before, how very precious life is.

If you or someone you know have been diagnosed with cancer it might help you to know that there is much that can be done to help you through it. The Cancer Journey is here to help guide you wherever you are on your own journey.

This book was written by three people each of whom has or has had cancer. At the time of writing, one of us was undergoing treatment after being diagnosed for the third time, one of us was dealing with a second diagnosis and pursuing alternative treatment and the third had recovered after the first diagnosis. We are enormously thankful for the medical support we have, and in addition to our conventional treatment we have all found that there is a lot we can do to help ourselves. This book is a fusion of our experiences and ideas and while we have all taken different routes, we have endeavoured to share the insights we have learned along the way.

> Everything in this book is our suggestion for you to cherry-pick as you go along. If something resonates with you, try it, if not, then don't. There is no right or wrong way to deal with a cancer diagnosis – do what works for you.

In the early stages of diagnosis it's not unusual to feel detached, which can stifle our ability to react to our situation in a constructive way. However, the good news is that we can learn to acknowledge and embrace the concerns of what our diagnosis means, and doing this can empower and motivate us to find new meaning in our lives.

In this book we will travel with you on your journey of cancer diagnosis, treatment and beyond so whether you're in the earliest stages or further along you will find help and advice that we hope will be useful to you.

We have all been fearful at one time but we have found paths to enable us to move forward and we want to help you learn how to overcome being overwhelmed and help you deal with your fear. Along the way we will give you the tools to help you live your life on your own terms and empower you to make decisions **with** your doctors, rather than just being a passenger on someone else's bus! We hope we can help guide you to take control of your wellbeing and lifestyle choices and ensure you increase your personal odds of recovery. And most importantly we want to share with you the comforting feeling that you are not alone on your journey.

Be prepared your life is going to change! That much is out of your hands. It's how you choose to deal with it that will make the difference.

Part 1
Your Diagnosis

.

Dealing With Your Diagnosis

CHAPTER 1

Dealing With Your Diagnosis – What We Wish We'd Been Told

The Initial Diagnosis

Being told that you have cancer is an intensely frightening experience. Although we all react in our own unique way, for most of us it brings an overwhelming and sickening fear and feels like our world is suddenly spiralling out of our control. Often the words, 'You have cancer' is the last clear thing you hear in that initial appointment because the rest of the conversation becomes a blur.

Our advice for this consultation would be to take someone with you who knows you very well. While you will want to put your hands over your ears like a child who doesn't want to hear what's being said and hope it will go away, they will hopefully assume responsibility for hearing what will happen next and make sure your needs are met as well as making sure you get home in one piece.

Knowing how to communicate your diagnosis to friends and family can be difficult so we have provided you with some suggestions in Chapter 4 that will give you some guidance.

Questions You May Want to Ask Your Doctor

1. What tests will I need?

2. When will tests/treatment start?

3. Is surgery/treatment absolutely necessary?

4. What are my treatment choices and what are the benefits/risks of each?

5. What is the success rate of treatment for this cancer?

6. Will I be admitted to hospital and if so for how long?

7. What side-effects can I expect on receiving treatment?

8. How long will treatment last?

9. Will I need to change my usual activities and if so for how long?

10. How closely will I be monitored and how often will scans take place?

11. How will I know if my treatment has worked?

12. Will my fertility be affected and if so can I harvest my eggs/sperm?

13. Is there anything I can do to prepare for treatment?

14. Can I get a second opinion?

15. Where can I get more information about my condition?

CHAPTER 2
How To Get The Best Out Of Your Doctors

Medical Support

The first thing to remember is the medical team looking after you is on your side! We have found that being polite and friendly paves the way to a better relationship with them. It can get out of hand though: Nick was blamed by the nurses on the chemo unit for them putting on weight because of the boxes of Krispy Kreme doughnuts which were brought in by a caring friend!

We understand how easy it is to take your frustrations out on the medical staff especially if they are administering an unpleasant procedure. We know it's stating the obvious but they have off days too and the occasional smile or even joke from you can make all the difference.

Your doctor/consultant has gone through years at medical school and additional years of learning their speciality. Let them know how much you value and appreciate their care and expertise. However, do remember that, while you may not be medically qualified, in many respects you know your body and history better than anyone else and it will be to your benefit to assert your role as the expert on you. Never be afraid to ask about the medication you are being given and why. It is your body after all. Polly was christened, 'Miss 24 questions' by her medical team owing to her inquisitive and challenging nature!

> Your future in your hands: Alongside the direction of your consultants, take as much responsibility as you are able to for your treatments.

Unfortunately, occasionally you meet a doctor who is lacking in people skills and who definitely has not kissed the Blarney Stone! So what can you do? Having a consultant who appears to be abrupt, aloof and uncommunicative was a predicament that one of us had to deal with. This was a particularly difficult situation as the consultant was renowned as being one of the top specialists in the country. Do you ask to be transferred to another specialist and hope they're as good? Or do you take on the task of educating someone who is lacking in interpersonal skills and hope you can improve the relationship? Despite feeling absolutely terrible because of the treatment, our patient liked a challenge so opted for the latter! Strategies employed included always being the first to extend a hand to shake his, asking open ended questions and using the journalists favourite tool of asking 'who, what, why, when and how' along with some subtle mirroring of body language. With time, things started to improve. If you are interested in discovering more about communication skills see the resources page. It is useful to remember to use the 'iron fist in a velvet glove' technique.

Be polite and gentle but firm.

Consultations

Learn as much as you can about your diagnosis from your GP, consultant and specialists but don't spend time researching on the internet unless directed to a particular site by your health care providers. A lot of internet information is misleading and you may come across 'quacks' trying to sell the promise of miraculous results. At the back of this book there is a resource page of organisations, websites of cancer charities, and books that we have found helpful that provide a balanced approach.

Whenever you have a consultation it is a good idea to write down a list of questions beforehand and if possible have someone with you to write down the answers. If you don't want anyone with you, take a tape recorder or mobile phone that has a voice recording facility and record the session. Be sure to ask the doctor's permission and explain it's so that you can take time to go over it and consider what has been said and not because you're going to take legal action against them!

Don't be afraid to ask for as much information as you need as the more you learn about your illness and the treatments available, the better able you are to make informed decisions and ask the right questions. You don't always get a second chance to ask questions so make the most of the time you have with your doctor. You may think you'll remember everything you're told but the chances are high that you won't, so always try to keep a record. Keeping notes for yourself can empower you and help you to better understand your condition and the possible options available for your treatment. One of the most powerful questions we've used is 'Doctor, what would you do if you were in my situation?' Don't be afraid to push for answers, but be prepared you might not always like what you hear. We know this from bitter experience!

A very important thing to remember when going to consultations, appointments or just about anywhere on your own, is to take a mobile phone with you and make sure it's charged up. We've had the experience of coming out of an appointment and bursting into tears and being unable to contact anyone. It's essential that you are able to contact someone for support, should you wish to.

> Always take a charged mobile phone with you.

Treatment

The 3 most common conventional treatments for cancer are surgery, chemotherapy and radiotherapy. **Chemotherapy** is treatment with anti-cancer drugs and **radiotherapy** is administration of carefully measured doses of radiation to kill the cancer cells.

If you need to have chemotherapy, there are a few practical things you may find useful.

If you're receiving chemotherapy via an intravenous drip involving a 6-7 hour process, you may want to wear your comfiest loose-fitting clothing like a tracksuit or leggings as lying or sitting in jeans is very restricting for your body. It's important to be comfortable allowing your body and skin to breathe. We found it helpful to wear a T-shirt underneath a cosy jumper for chemo days so that accessing the forearm or wrist is easier for inserting the drip.

A fortunate few manage to sail through chemo feeling fairly well but just tired. However, for many, the most common and unpleasant side effects of chemotherapy are nausea and vomiting and unfortunately these often come with either diarrhoea or constipation. Fortunately there are lots of antidotes available and your healthcare team will do whatever they can to minimise any side-effects. However, if you do suffer you can also help yourself by preparing some anti-sickness solutions. We have provided some suggestions in our Recipe section in Chapter 11.

Because the treatment is a long process, you might want to take along a book to read, a crossword puzzle book or a portable device which allows you to listen to music or watch movies to help fill the time. To help you relax you could download a meditation CD to let you access your inner calm during the treatment. Take a healthy snack such as fruit or muesli bars in case you get hungry, and remember to take water with you and drink plenty throughout.

If you're receiving radiotherapy, again we would recommend you wear your comfiest loose-fitting clothing so you can slip in and out of it easily, ready for treatment. Ladies, you might want to invest in a sports-bra to wear (with no metal in it) for scan days to avoid flashing anything from behind those pesky loose-fitting hospital robes!

We know only too well that on occasion the machines can break down meaning your timeslot for treatment gets pushed back and there can be a lot of waiting around.

> After becoming grumpy and irritable when he had to wait an age for chemotherapy, a friend made Nick laugh when he said, 'That's why it's called a Waiting Room. The sign on the door doesn't read Fast-track Room!'

Take advantage of the time to read a book or magazine, meditate or write while you're waiting. You know better than most that time is precious so actively decide to make the most of it. Once again, take snacks and water with you so you don't end up buying something unhealthy from the tuck machine or hospital canteen.

If you're lucky enough to get to choose what time you have your scans, you may want to pick an early morning slot to avoid having to fast all day. Not all scans require you to have an empty stomach but some do.

The Cancer Journey

/

CHAPTER 3

Side Effects

Depending on which treatment(s) you undergo, it is likely you will experience one or more side-effects. We have listed a few of them along with some suggestions as to how to overcome them or at least help to manage them.

> It helps to remind yourself that this too shall pass!

Constipation and Diarrhoea

Anyone know a good plumber? During treatment, you may experience either constipation or diarrhoea. If you're really lucky, you'll get both! Normally, chemotherapy brings the gift of constipation making you feel and look like the Michelin Man. This is caused by the chemotherapy drugs which can numb the nerves in the bowel and may continue to affect you even once treatment has halted. Anti-sickness drugs and painkillers can sometimes make this worse.

If you are suffering from **constipation**, there are a number of things you can do:

- Eat more fibre such as fruits, vegetables, brown rice and linseed (otherwise known as flaxseed). Eat dried fruits such as apricots, figs and of course prunes.

- Drink more fluids – you should be consuming at least 2 litres of water a day and can top this up by drinking herbal teas, freshly made juices, prune juice and homemade soups.

- As detailed in Chapter 10, we recommend you avoid eating foods high in fat and sugar such as sweets and processed foods. These will also aggravate constipation so do your best to treat them as the cancer fertilizer they are and steer well clear.

- We would advise a natural approach to counteracting constipation rather than laxatives, especially as they can cause cramping, gas, bloating and diarrhoea.

If you have **diarrhoea** the most important thing to do is prevent dehydration. Drink plenty of fluids but stay away from caffeinated drinks and alcohol. Drinks such as ginger ale or carrot juice are good but don't drink fruit juices as they may make the condition worse. In general a clear liquid diet is recommended such as chicken broth or clear soups and blackberry or ginger tea which can all help. If you do feel like eating, go gently on your system.

We recommend the BRAT diet. No, this isn't just for kids (although it is recommended for children with diarrhoea) – it stands for bananas, rice, apples and toast. With diarrhoea your body becomes depleted of potassium and bananas are an excellent source of this and they're also easily digestible, easy to eat and nutritious. Brown rice contains vitamins B_1 and B_3 and iron. Apples should be cooked or baked as this process softens the cellulose which then helps to absorb water in the bowel. Avoid milk and dairy products including ice cream but do eat probiotic yoghurt as the active cultures in this can help with the symptoms and replace the naturally occurring bacteria that our system needs.

See Recipes in Chapter 11 for more information.

For those days when you feel like you've had enough and you can't go on – don't despair!

10 things to help you get through a dark day

1. If being left alone suits you, turn off your mobile phone and any forms of communication!

2. If it's better for you to have company, ask an understanding friend to come over and support you.

3. Commit to venturing no further than the distance between your bed and the kitchen.

4. Make yourself something comforting to drink and eat, for example, Banana Ice Cream or warm Almond Milk (see Chapter 11).

5. Go back to bed and put on a movie & watch it while snuggling under the duvet.

6. Nap.

7. Stick your head out of the window and breathe in fresh air.

8. Return to bed.

9. Watch another movie

10. Sleep for 8 hours as tomorrow will be a better day!

Nausea and Vomiting

Nausea and vomiting can be caused by the cancer itself; by prescribed treatments i.e., chemotherapy, radiotherapy, surgery or may even be brought on by the anxiety you feel about the disease or its treatment. In the case of the latter it's not uncommon to have 'anticipatory' nausea or vomiting. This is where the memory of a previous episode of nausea or vomiting is enough to trigger another bout – possibly when you're going for a repeat treatment.

Fortunately, as well as the many anti-sickness (antiemetic) drugs available there are some things you can do to help yourself. We would recommend the following;

- Don't force yourself to eat but make absolutely sure you keep up your fluid intake. It's essential you don't become dehydrated.

- Sip clear cold drinks such as iced water. Some people find fizzy drinks such as ginger beer or lemonade help to quell the nausea, although do try other alternatives first as we aren't huge fans of fizzy drinks thanks to the dangerous aspartame that they often contain.

- Herbal teas such as peppermint and ginger may help.

- Nausea tends to be worse on an empty stomach so do try to eat small snacks or meals throughout the day.

- Ginger biscuits and peppermints can both suppress nausea.

- Avoid preparing or eating food that has a strong smell.

- Eat slowly and rest well afterwards but don't lie flat.

- If you can, take a walk in the fresh air as this can help with nausea and may also stimulate a poor appetite.

- Avoid wearing tight fitting clothes.

- Meditation and visualisation can help with nausea and vomiting (see Chapter 6).

- Acupuncture and acupressure have also been shown to be effective against nausea and vomiting (see Chapter 7).

- Travel wrist bands (seabands) which are available from chemists use the same principle as acupressure. By applying pressure to the specific points on the wrist, nausea is hopefully controlled.

Lymphoedema

Lymphoedema is the build-up of lymph fluid in soft body tissues and can occur as a result of cancer or after surgery or radiation treatment. It often happens when the lymph system is damaged or blocked e.g. when lymph nodes have been removed.

Post-treatment, two of us suffered from lymphoedema. Polly had severe swelling in one leg to the point where walking was really difficult and at times terribly painful. On visiting a lymphoedema clinic, she was told that there was no cure and that she would have to 'learn to live with it'. The gauntlet was down. Polly duly informed the nurse that this prospect was unacceptable and that alternative means would be tried. By adopting a positive attitude, and using visualisation, meditation, manual lymphatic drainage (see overleaf) and gratitude for its healing, while eating healthily and juicing, the lymphoedema began to reduce. Over the course of the following visits to the clinic, the lymphoedema nurse was astounded and admitted the circumference of the leg had reduced dramatically in size and, to this day, there is very little difference in size between Polly's legs. Reiterating what we said earlier – you know your body best. Don't let anyone dictate to you what you are or are not capable of doing.

Pam also suffered with quite severe lymphoedema but in her back – on one side from waist to shoulder blade. The only solution offered was surgical aspiration which has associated risks of infection (a sterile needle is inserted to draw off the excess fluid). Again dissension stepped into place and Pam declined the procedure in preference to trying to solve the problem by more natural means. After just one week of many daily simple lymphatic drainage massage movements the fluid had significantly reduced. And after three weeks virtually all signs of lymphoedema had disappeared.

Manual Lymphatic Drainage (MLD) is an advanced massage therapy in which the practitioner uses a range of specialised and very light rhythmic pumping massage techniques to move the lymph fluid, which is located just under the skin. This stimulates the lymphatic vessels which carry substances vital to the defence of the body in the direction of the lymph nodes or glands, which contain cells that fight infection and get rid of waste and bacteria. MLD is used to treat and control different types of lymphoedema and relieves fluid congestion anywhere in the body where there is an abnormal build-up of lymph fluid. As it is a very specialised technique, it should only be given by a trained therapist, but it is possible for an individual to be taught a simplified method called Simple Lymphatic Drainage (SLD) so that you can treat yourself at home.

Your lymphoedema nurse or physiotherapist should be able to teach you SLD but if you have trouble finding someone suitably qualified you can contact MLD UK who can provide a register of their members. As well as stimulating the immune system and being an important treatment for lymphoedema, MLD is also very relaxing and may help to improve your sleeping patterns and any restlessness you may be experiencing.

We can, therefore, attest to the fact that there are alternative ways to counter lymphoedema without surgical intervention but you may need professional help to facilitate them.

Another technique which is worth trying is **dry skin brushing**. This practice increases circulation to the skin and greatly aids lymphatic drainage of the entire body. All you need is a long-handled body brush with natural bristles or it can be done with a loofah. It should be carried out on dry skin and we recommend you do it daily first thing in the morning to jump start your circulation. It's also preferable to do it prior to your shower or bath so that the dead skin cells are washed away.

The technique is simple. Begin brushing your bare skin in long sweeping strokes from your feet upwards, brushing the legs, buttocks then onto the stomach and chest. Brush from the hands towards the shoulders and from the waist up your back, brushing several times in each area, over-lapping as you go. Always brush towards the heart and avoid sensitive areas and anywhere the skin is broken.

Brushing your body in this way every day is a very simple and effective way of encouraging your body's discharge of metabolic waste and excess fluid, thus supporting your other eliminative organs such as the kidneys and liver as well as improving your skin tone.

Insomnia

It is estimated that between 30-50% of people with cancer experience insomnia. This can be caused by pain, the cancer itself or cancer-related drug treatment, as well as the very normal psychological impact of anxiety-related sleep disturbance. It is not unusual for a patient to view insomnia as a much lesser issue than their cancer diagnosis and therefore not raise it with their doctors, particularly if they are overwhelmed by other problems such as chemotherapy, radiotherapy, nausea or pain. But it can, nevertheless, have an immense negative impact on quality of life and can significantly decrease your ability to function and cope. Additionally it can increase other symptoms such as fatigue and anxiety, and it can also decrease the cancer patient's tolerance of pain.

While your doctor can prescribe sleep medications, we have found a variety of simple self-help techniques that are effective in managing insomnia and have described a couple of exercises that you may find helpful. Even if they don't immediately send you into a deep sleep, they will hopefully help you achieve a lovely restful state and this in itself will be beneficial.

Try to follow a calming bedtime routine involving quiet, soothing activities rather than anything stimulating or energetic. Taking a warm bath and having a glass of warm milk or a cup of soothing chamomile tea before bed can help induce relaxation (alcohol should be avoided).

The following exercises may help;

Deep Breathing: Lie on your back with your hands either resting on your abdomen or by your sides with your shoulders relaxed. Start by exhaling fully so that your lungs are empty. Now slowly take in a deep breath through your nose and as you do this be aware of expanding your lungs, stomach and ribcage. As you release the breath, let your abdomen slowly return to its original place. Continue to do this for 10 breaths counting each inhalation and exhalation as you go, constantly being aware of the movement of your ribcage. If your mind wanders off and you lose count, don't worry. Just refocus on your counting and continue to follow this cycle of deep breathing until you fall asleep.

If you find it difficult to lie on your back, lie on your side and breathe through your mouth rather than your nose.

Progressive Muscle Relaxation: This technique is again best done while lying flat on your back but, if this is not comfortable, lie on your side. With each deep breath in, you will tense a muscle group, hold for a count of 5 and then release the hold while exhaling. By alternately tensing and relaxing each muscle group in a sequential pattern from toes to head, you will release all tension from your body and at the end should feel very relaxed and sleepy.

Take a deep breath in and tense your toes as tightly as you can and hold for a count of 5, then release the hold and exhale slowly. Take another deep breath and flex your toes upwards, feeling the muscles in your calves tightening. Hold for a count of 5 then relax and exhale. Squeeze your thighs together and clench your buttocks, hold then release. Suck in your stomach as you inhale, hold for a count of 5 then release. Stretch your back and neck, making yourself as long as possible, hold then release. Shrug up your shoulders towards your ears, feeling the tension in your upper arms as well. Hold then let go. Clench your hands making tight fists and feel the muscles in your lower arms also contracting, hold, then release. Scrunch up your face, squeezing your eyelids tightly shut, hold for 5, then let go.

By the time you have worked your way up to the top of your body you should feel deeply relaxed and calm, and the effort and concentration involved in the exercise should also leave you feeling tired and ready for a deep sleep.

These exercises can also be useful if you waken during the night and find it difficult to get back to sleep.

Other techniques that you could try are meditation or visualisation, and we have given more details of these in Chapter 6. You could also try listening to soothing music or relaxation CDs.

Night Sweats

Night sweats can be a side effect of cancer medications and they can also be a symptom of certain kinds of cancer (especially lymphomas). They can add profoundly to your existing stress by interrupting your sleep, making you uncomfortable and frustrated and generally decreasing the quality of your life. It occurs because either the disease or the medication causes confusion in the thermal regulation of the body.

Acupuncture (see Chapter 7) has been shown to be effective in treating night sweats for some people and there are also a number of very simple practical steps you can take. Keep the bedroom cool and have a fan and iced water by the bed to help ease any episodes. Wear cotton night clothes and use a number of layers of cotton bedding. You can then shed some layers if you get hot during the night but leave enough to keep you comfortable. Also avoid eating spicy food and drinking caffeine or alcohol; these all have the potential to raise your blood sugar level which may trigger more episodes. Drinking herbal teas such as sage or chamomile have also been reported to be helpful as well as taking vitamin E supplements.

Restless Leg Syndrome

Restless legs are thought to be caused by a deficiency in magnesium, B vitamins or iron. They can also be a symptom of poor kidney function or as a side effect of some drugs. You will usually experience uncomfortable or unpleasant sensations in your legs accompanied by an urge to move them. In fact, it's virtually impossible not to move them! Occasionally the arms are affected too. Symptoms are often worse during periods of inactivity or rest and hence are most likely to occur in the evening particularly when you're trying to get to sleep. Very frustratingly they can also wake you during the night and leave you feeling exhausted the next day. The symptoms are usually eased by stretching, moving, walking or massaging the legs. The severity can also be reduced by doing some gentle stretching exercise like yoga or Pilates and taking a warm bath before bed.

You could also try eating (or juicing) foods that are rich in the vitamins and minerals in which you may be deficient. Some suggestions would be magnesium and iron rich green foods such as spinach, watercress, broccoli and kale as well as berries, beetroot, citrus fruit, fennel and peppers. If symptoms persist, you could ask your doctor for an appropriate supplement.

Caffeine is thought to aggravate the condition so we would advise you cut all forms of this out of your diet. To give you a leg up (excuse the pun!) we have given you a hearty juice in the Recipe section (Chapter 11) which we hope will give your legs a rest.

Oral Thrush

Oral thrush is caused by a fungus called Candida. While this fungus is present naturally in most of the population, it only becomes a problem when there's a change in the chemistry of the mouth, which favours Candida over the other naturally occurring micro-organisms that are present. These changes are not uncommon in people undergoing chemotherapy or taking medications such as steroids or antibiotics. They can also occur in people with an immune deficiency or with poor nutrition. Thrush normally appears as white or cream coloured spots or patches on the tongue or inside the cheeks or throat. The infected area may bleed when scraped, give a burning sensation and you may also get discomfort when chewing or swallowing food.

Normal treatment is with prescribed antifungal medicines but you can also help the condition yourself. A good oral hygiene routine is really important but thrush can make your mouth so sensitive that normal brushing is impossible. Try to use a very soft toothbrush and regularly rinse your mouth with warm salt water. Your doctor or a pharmacist can also recommend an appropriate mouth wash.

Candida is systemic and can be tricky to eradicate, especially as a standard UK diet provides the ideal environment for it to thrive. We recommend taking good quality probiotics and incorporating fermented foods (See Chapter 10) into your diet to help restore the balance of good intestinal bacteria and help reduce sweet food cravings. Avoid refined carbohydrates such as white bread, white rice, pasta and sugary foods such as cakes and biscuits. Also try to minimise the amount of cows' products such as milk, butter and cheese as they can aggravate the condition. Instead try sheep, goat, rice, coconut or nut milk. Go for a high fibre diet and eat unsweetened, full fat live probiotic yoghurt, which will help counter the fungus.

If you have cancer, it's almost certain that you already have or are likely to develop Candida so we recommend reading Donna Gates' *The*

Body Ecology Diet which will help you get a better understanding of how to tackle it. See Resources Section for more information.

Dry Mouth

Chemotherapy and radiotherapy can both cause a dry mouth. Particularly with treatments for the head and neck area; saliva glands can become damaged and less productive. This can make eating and swallowing difficult so try to go for liquid foods such as soups, stews and noodle dishes and accompany meals with sauces and gravies. Snack on celery sticks and cucumber which both have high water content as this can help stimulate the saliva glands and add moisture to your mouth. While sipping a drink doesn't always help, we have found that sucking on an ice lolly sometimes does (see Chapter 11 for recipes).

Cramps

Muscle cramps can be caused by muscle fatigue, dehydration, low blood magnesium (sometimes associated with cancer therapy) or sudden changes in temperature. They can also be caused by electrolyte disturbance such as low levels of calcium, magnesium and potassium. Almost all cancer therapies can cause you to feel fatigued and electrolyte imbalance is a known side effect of chemotherapy. If you're unfortunate enough to be suffering from night sweats also, the chances are you'll be dehydrated, have low blood salt (through excessive sweating) and also suffer from sudden changes in temperature. For people dealing with cancer treatment the chances of having cramp are, therefore, very high.

The most common areas to get cramp are the feet (almost bearable), calves (painful) and hamstrings (agony) – the bigger the muscle the greater the pain! And the most usual time to get cramp is during the night.

The good news is there are a number of self-help remedies. Although you probably won't feel like it if you're tired, it can really help to go for a walk before going to bed. This will both stretch and strengthen the muscles. It can also help to drink water before bedtime to make sure you're well hydrated. Although this might mean getting up to go to the loo in the night, the extra exercise may also minimise the chance of getting cramps. It can also help to sleep with a pillow under your knees. During the day try to increase your fluid intake (non-caffeinated, non-alcoholic drinks) and make sure you get plenty of magnesium, calcium and potassium into your diet. Foods such as apple, apricot, banana, blueberry, blackcurrant, cherry, kiwi, melon, nectarine and orange contain all three minerals. Some of the vegetables that also contain these are beetroot, carrot, cucumber, fennel and pepper.

If you prefer to take medication, your doctor can also prescribe quinine sulphate tablets but drinking tonic water which contains quinine will have the same effect.

Things that may relieve the cramping include moving, rubbing and stretching the affected area and taking a hot shower or bath i.e. anything which increases blood flow to the muscles.

CHAPTER 4

Communication

Breaking the News – Distress Management

Initially, it's unlikely to be obvious to anyone else that you have had this diagnosis, so it's up to you to decide who should be made aware of your situation and how soon. But even if you initially choose to hide it from the world at large, do try to share it with someone close to you as, dealing with this on your own, can be a very isolating and frightening experience. However, on the other hand, be wary of being sucked into telling everyone about your situation and replaying the drama over and over again. It is very easy to fall into the trap where you talk about it so much and reassure loved ones by saying 'I'm really okay' that you eventually subconsciously separate yourself from how you *really* feel. Also, the more people you talk to, the more you are likely to involve yourself in how upset they are for you and this can be exhausting.

> Breaking the news – be aware that others may not react as you expect. Help them, support them but don't let their reactions suppress your needs.

It's difficult to predict how those close to you will react to your illness. Within your immediate family the dynamics can be delicate and it's important to try not to place expectations on others. Some people will step forward and others will step back, and it may take time to understand what support others are able and comfortable to give (also see Chapter 9: What Family and Friends can do to Help). It's easy to fall into a pattern of focusing on yourself and your current state, but remember that being the loved one of a person with a life-threatening illness is very stressful and can even be excruciating at times. Showing love, compassion and appreciation for those supporting you can be quite a powerful counter to our own feelings of helplessness.

Telling Your Children

We found that the best thing is to tell your offspring as soon as possible after your diagnosis. This has two benefits; the first being that you don't ruminate on it endlessly which will save you enormous stress and, secondly if you don't tell them they will pick up on your stress anyway and you can save them from thinking they've done something wrong or imagining something even worse. As a parent you know your child better than anyone else, and we recommend you trust and believe in your own intuition on how and what to tell them. This won't be easy and will need careful thought and a bit of planning. There are useful organisations such as Macmillan Cancer Support who can help you through this difficult process.

If you are able it's usually best to break the news to them yourself. If possible having your partner with you and maybe also grandparents or other close relatives who may be involved with childcare will also be really helpful. If they hear it from someone else, your children's imagination may run wild sending them into a panic, or they may feel isolated or not important enough to be told firsthand.

Try to keep the explanation simple and appropriate for their age and also be honest but remember you don't need to tell them everything all at once. It's important to prepare them for what's going to happen in the immediate term, and reassure them they'll be loved and cared for even if you're in hospital or too unwell. Also encourage them to ask questions and be as honest as you can with the answers, but don't push them to talk if they don't want to. If they ask something which you feel unable or unwilling to explain it's better to tell them you don't know the answer at the moment, rather than make something up just to reassure them. Let them know that you appreciate their feelings and that's it OK for them to be upset while also encouraging them to support your efforts to think positively.

> You may be amazed at how resilient and supportive kids can be!

Pam was made to smile on coming home after surgery. A lovely little bunch of pink, red and blue flowers had been freshly picked by her young daughter and placed beside the bed with the question, 'Do you like the flowers, Mummy – I picked them so they would match?'. As the bedroom carpet was a purple colour Pam replied, 'Yes they're lovely! Did you pick them to match the carpet?' 'No' came the reply, 'I picked them to match your bruises!'

For some of us it can be very helpful to have group therapy and to be able to talk openly about our feelings with others in a similar situation. Family and friends can sometimes find talking about the potential prognosis morbid, and may downplay the seriousness of your illness as they cannot cope with it. This can make you feel you have to protect their feelings and can result in you feeling alone and even resentful. Group therapy can provide a unique opportunity to vent emotions as well as sharing knowledge of treatments and therapies. Apart from helping you to feel less isolated, providing concrete empathetic support to other group members, often gives a unique opportunity to enhance our own self esteem.

While some people benefit from group therapy others find the very thought of it an anathema and prefer something much less formal. Chatting to somebody else who is going through similar experiences to you over a cup of tea can be a great help. There are organisations that run drop-in centres where you can do a variety of activities and these can be useful in combating isolation. The important thing is to maintain contact with other people be it friends, family or other cancer patients.

Let Email Do The Work For You

It can be really draining repeating how you are feeling over and over again, but try to remember that those who ask really do want to know because they care about you. Sending a round robin email is an excellent way of keeping in touch. We know you've probably groaned about those Christmas emails from people gloating how their wonderful children are getting top grades and the fabulous holidays etc. But this is different; you have a serious illness and people will be glad they are able to communicate with you via email. By doing this you are able to get your news out without going insane having to repeat yourself! You can also use email to suggest to family and friends how they can help you by advising others when ready for visitors.

Here's an example of what you could write;

Dear all,

Thank you all for your lovely messages – it is amazing to know I have such a wonderful support system.

As some of you may already know, it has been confirmed by my doctor that I have cancer.

He/She has told me that it is very treatable and has recommended radiotherapy/chemotherapy/surgery which will begin on [insert date].

OR

He/She has told me that treatment is not possible and has therefore suggested we monitor my health over the next six months while I make changes to my diet and lifestyle which can improve my overall health. I have been told the prognosis is good/not good. However I have absolute faith that I will beat this. There are so many other things that I can do to boost my chances and with your love and support, I will do so. During my treatment I have been told to expect to feel [nauseous/tired/ run down]. I would really love someone to accompany me to hospital over this time should anyone want to be my 'chemo buddy'! Maybe someone could organise a schedule as I will be having treatment over a 3/6/9 week period?

(Disclaimer: as my chemo buddy you agree to hold my hair back while I worship the porcelain god, feed me grapes, make me laugh and remind me that ordinary life is waiting for me to get back to it!)

It would also be hugely helpful if anyone could kindly collect the children from school on those dates. I hope to feel well enough to continue at work but until I begin treatment, it is very difficult to know how I'm going to feel.

I am going to do everything within my power to beat this and look forward to celebrating with you all on getting an 'all clear' from my doctors in the very near future!

With love xx

> Don't describe yourself as a cancer 'victim'. Take an empowered stance: the moment you are diagnosed, you are a cancer survivor!

The following is a text message that Polly sent to work colleagues and friends on her diagnosis:

Hi everyone,

Some of you may know that I have been having tests lately which have unfortunately confirmed that I have cancer once again in my lymph nodes. My doctor has recommended radiotherapy so I will be going under the radar for the foreseeable. Please don't be offended if I don't return your emails, calls or texts – I really do appreciate them – I just need some time to myself and take this opportunity to thank you all in advance for love and support.

Xx

Although Polly chose not to have treatment this text message allowed her the space and time to come to this decision without the pressure or concerns of others.

Often visitors don't come prepared to keep the conversation going, and it's hard enough for us just getting through the day without having to put on a cabaret act. When Nick was in an isolation ward he got very cheeky and suggested that visitors brought two pieces of gossip *a la* OK magazine and if they didn't know any to make it up! This led to some hilarious and outrageous tales leading to roars of laughter. We definitely recommend you try it.

> ### Foot-In-Mouth Prevention
> Friends and loved ones, please don't ask how long the doctor has 'given me'! And please don't throw me a pity party! Show your concern but treat me as you normally would.

The Cancer Journey

CHAPTER 5

Taking Care of Your Emotional Needs

Your Psyche

Cancer is one of those things that happen in our lives that we have no control over. We regard these type of events as catastrophes yet in the long term they may also turn out to be positive and beneficial experiences. We are always amazed at the number of people who are able to use having cancer as a life enhancing experience rather than a catastrophe.

> It's not what happens; it's how we react to it that matters.

Having cancer is not what they would have chosen for themselves, but the realisation that they have a choice in how they react is very empowering. Research continues to document that a positive attitude can boost our immune system and therefore increase our ability to fight illness.

Philosopher and author Professor John Gray says, '…in everyday life we do not scan our options beforehand, then enact the one that is best. We simply deal with whatever is at hand'. If this is so and we just act and react, then it makes sense to review the actions we have taken each day to be aware of the consequences and take note to see if they are helping or hindering us. Being overwhelmed and feeling vulnerable are natural reactions. The key is to take time to mentally and emotionally process all you are going through and then try to plan your coping strategy in as positive a way as possible. Mentally make the shift from the negative (having cancer) to the positive (treatment and recovery).

Make sure you allow yourself plenty of extra time when doing things, and remember you are dealing with a major illness – some days it will take all your effort to just get out of bed! Try to accept the situation as it is rather than mentally resisting it.

Inner Strength

As you progress with your treatment there will be times when you will feel you can't go on. You may have lost your hair, felt nauseous, had fatigue like you never thought possible, and, as for constipation – what would you give for your bowels to be working normally (it seems that with many cancer treatments it's all or nothing – constipation or diarrhoea)! So it should come as no surprise that you feel irritable and frustrated which often results in losing your temper with the unfortunate checkout assistant or your partner over the most trivial thing. You're at the end of your tether and the frustration seems to grow and grow driving home the message…if only…what's the point, and finally, why me? The frustration and helplessness you feel is because you are experiencing a loss of your life and identity. You are unable to do many of the things you used to do, and your physical appearance may have been changed either from surgery or chemotherapy. But remember, there are still a lot of things you can do and enjoy if you only stop and think about it. To quote John Diamond in his book *C: Because Cowards Get Cancer Too*, 'Cancer is a word, it is not a sentence.'

And perhaps when we are having one of those days, it's the perfect opportunity to discover deep within us our own inner strength and that place where resilience is born. The resilience that will give you the power to say, "I choose to live my life to the full regardless of how I feel and what my prognosis may be". Discovering your own inner strength can be like being born again, giving you the freedom to make choices and take decisions that in the past might have seemed impossible.

> Say YES to life!

Having that new sense of inner strength can liberate us to be able to be who we want to be. Going through the experience of having cancer is obviously not one you would have chosen but, as it is happening, know that you are left with a choice. You can either feel sorry for yourself or look within yourself and confront the demons that may be limiting you now or have done so in the past. Doing this gives us confidence. You may find you still feel apprehensive about trying new things but living through this experience you have a reference point. We have probably faced what we feared most which was to have cancer and are now discovering that being able to deal with this, we are capable of facing just about anything.

During your cancer treatment you will experience a wide range of emotions. Be prepared for this and accept they will happen, but try not to shout at the traffic warden or bus driver! Even though things may seem difficult, it can be extremely useful to keep a gratitude journal to make a note of those things in your life that you are grateful for. Now you might think we have gone completely bonkers suggesting this. You're probably reading this thinking, 'I have cancer, what have I got to be thankful for?' Psychologists are finding that people who practise gratitude don't suffer from depression as much as those who don't practice. If you have never tried it, it's worth a go as you have enough to deal with without adding depression to the list. Professor Richard Wiseman in his book *59 Seconds* says, 'Expressing gratitude, thinking about a perfect future and affectionate writing has been scientifically proven to work.' So it makes sense to try it out and see for yourself. You might say to yourself, 'I know that cancer has taken lots from me, but it has also given me a strength and courage I didn't know I had and a much deeper appreciation for my family and friends, and for this I really am grateful'.

At the end of your treatment, apart from the enormous relief of finishing, an emotion that sometimes comes up unexpectedly is how quickly family and friends are to resume their normal lives and leave you feeling somewhat abandoned. Try not to take this as a lack of caring on their part. Like you, they have probably been under a lot of stress and focused a lot of their energy on supporting you, and they also will be relieved that your treatment is completed but they now need to replenish their own energy supplies. Try to be compassionate towards them and share your gratitude for their support.

Loss

A diagnosis of cancer comes with many, many losses most of which have associated fears, but with these can come extraordinary opportunities. If we choose to embrace and understand our illness it empowers us to face our fear and awakens us to live more fully. There's great loss from letting go of the things that illness takes away such as control of our lives, independence, self-worth, identity and self-esteem. You lose your naïve belief that you're immortal and that time is an unlimited resource. From this we can learn to question what and who are really important to us, and this can bring about a massive change in priorities. Fear can be a good motivator to start something new. But fear must gradually be replaced with the desire to enhance the quality of our lives.

> On the flip side of loss you have now gained exemption (probably temporary) from the eternal race to prove/improve yourself!

You are no longer forced to do or be what others expect of you, and you can live your life more authentically on your own terms.

Grief

When we lose something as major as our health, another natural emotional response is grief.

Elisabeth Kübler-Ross, M.D., was a Swiss-born psychiatrist and the author of the groundbreaking book *On Death and Dying*. Actively involved within the Hospice movement, in 1972 she developed what has come to be known as the five stages of grief. These are **Denial, Anger, Bargaining, Depression and Acceptance**. We feel we must stress that the stages of grief are only a model of behaviour, and as we are all unique individuals we will experience and react to situations differently, and therefore these stages are not necessarily the reality for everyone.

Kübler-Ross was a highly skilled therapist who became aware of these stages while working with people with life threatening illnesses. She held the belief that while not everyone will experience all of the stages of grief, the majority will experience at least two or more stages. From our experience we feel that knowledge of these stages can help us to understand the roller coaster of emotions that we live through while coming to terms with our illness. Realising that these feelings are normal helps regain a sense of control, reducing our feelings of isolation and vulnerability, leaving us better equipped to cope.

We like this quote from Dr Kübler-Ross, 'The ultimate lesson all of us have to learn is unconditional love, which includes not only others but ourselves as well.'

The Five Stages of Grief:

Denial

Once the initial shock of diagnosis has worn off, denial is a common reaction. It has been suggested that denial might be seen as the brain's way of protecting the body and mind from unbearable anxiety. While it may help some people deal with situations that appear too traumatic to face, it can also encourage an escape into fantasy. This is where we tell ourselves all kinds of stories, such as 'they've got it wrong' or 'I need a second opinion' believing the doctor has made a mistake. There may be times when a second opinion can be helpful but please discuss it with your GP or health visitor.

In cases of extreme classical denial it is not unusual to imagine there hasn't been a diagnosis at all. So, by continuing to live as though nothing has happened, or becoming compulsive in adopting a 'super' health regime we can convince our self we are fit and healthy. Therefore, the diagnosis must have been wrong. As difficult as it can be it is important to embrace the reality of the situation. Certainly, denial may give us a few moments to catch our breath, but ultimately we have to acknowledge our disease along with the treatments and interventions that go with it. So denial is only a temporary defence, and as it begins to fade all the feelings you were denying begin to surface.

Anger

The next stage after denial is usually anger, which comes when we accept we can no longer deny the diagnosis. Underneath anger is a sense of limitless pain. The expression of emotion associated with anger is like an outpouring of bottled-up feelings and frustrations that are often experienced as unexpected outbursts of rage, resentment and envy, extending to anyone close by, including your loved ones and strangers.

Our anger is often fuelled by a sense of how unfair it all is, and the question 'why me?' being repeated like an endless mantra in our minds. Although extremely uncomfortable for you and those close to you, remember that this is a natural response to what is, after all, a horrible injustice to you.

When you find yourself getting angry it can be useful to try an exercise that is often used in drama schools to access emotions. Take yourself somewhere you can be alone and have a good rant out loud about how unfair life is. If you find it difficult to do this, you could just try repeating out loud 'It's not fair that I have cancer. It's not fair I have cancer'. Keep going, listing all the different reasons why it is unfair and hopefully you will be all 'angered out'. Of course, we're not suggesting this is a 'happy pill' which will make all of your negative emotions suddenly disappear but you might find you get the first glimpse of acceptance and the wisdom in the Buddha's first noble truth that, '*Life is suffering.*'

Another exercise that has proven to be helpful is to write an anger journal putting the words and sentiments that express your sense of injustice and lack of fairness down on paper. Or perhaps combine it with a gratitude diary spending half the session expressing anger and the other half expressing gratitude for the good things and yes – there are always things in our lives to be grateful for, no matter how bad things may seem.

Bargaining

Bargaining is usually the negotiation with a higher power for us to gain time or have a lesser diagnosis in exchange for us doing good deeds or reforming our character in some way. 'Please God, I'll do/give anything if you let me have a few more years/let me live to see my children finish school', etc, etc. We are seeking in vain for a way out, or even just a postponement of the pain that we believe is ahead of us.

Bargaining is often accompanied by guilt and this can often make us angry with ourselves. 'If only I had gone to the doctor sooner.' 'If only I'd done x, y or z differently'.

Bargaining has been described as an expression of hope that the bad news may be reversible. It is not surprising to see people with illness turning to religion for solace. Others pursue soothsayers, healers and unfortunately questionable therapists peddling their wares – for which sadly too many people have been misled while making huge financial sacrifices in the hope of redemption and health.

Depression

The first thing we need to realise is that depression following a diagnosis of a life threatening illness is a normal and appropriate emotion. Having tried bargaining to no avail, our attention may now move more easily into reality and the present situation. Asking the question, 'Is there any point in carrying on?'. We may then not realise that we've become silent, withdrawn and intensely sad as we unconsciously begin the descent into depression. This is also very painful for those close to us and not something that can be snapped out of easily.

For all concerned it's also really important to realise this is not a sign of mental illness. It is just a natural stage in the grieving process of adapting to and accepting a future with different dreams and experiences than perhaps we had hoped for. Take comfort in the knowledge that this will pass, even though it may feel as though it will last forever and professional help will also really help.

If you are concerned that you are depressed please discuss it with you GP or your medical team as they can help you through this part of the process. But please let them know as soon as possible how you are feeling and that you need their help.

An exercise which may help with depression that you can do yourself comes from Cognitive Behaviour Therapy (CBT). CBT is a type of therapy that helps you manage your problems by changing how you think about yourself, the world and other people (cognitive) and how what you do affects your thoughts and feelings (behaviour). The exercise which we think you might find useful is called 'mood mapping'. Mood mapping helps us work out how we are feeling and what has triggered these feelings. We can then take practical steps to address when our mood is low.

The exercise is based on the principle that mood has two components, namely how much energy you have and how positive or negative you are feeling. You start by dividing a page into 4 quarters by drawing a vertical line representing your energy levels – top being high and bottom being low, crossed by a horizontal line – left being negative and right being positive. The four quarters represent your four basic moods;

- Top right quarter with high energy and feeling positive (action).

- Top left with high energy but feeling negative (stressed or anxious).

- Bottom left with low energy and feeling negative (depressed or exhausted).

- Bottom right with low energy but feeling positive (calm).

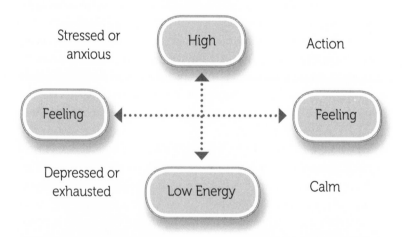

By plotting your feelings several times a day and keeping notes of what has contributed to how you feel you can easily identify the physical and emotional triggers for your mood. You can then take practical steps to do more of the positive and less of the negative things to keep your mood and life more stabilised.

Acceptance

When we finally arrive at acceptance it is like the dawning of a new day. It allows us to finally let go and stop struggling with ourselves. Acceptance is simply acknowledging the way things are, and to do other than this just puts us back into struggle and robs us of a sense of peace.

> Life is what it is and what is happening is what's happening. We can choose to feel miserable about it or not, but being miserable isn't going to change the situation – it's just going to make us feel miserable!

Making the emotional transition from diagnosis to acceptance is a voyage of discovery and one that we all take in one form or another. It will be a journey that some of us will repeat daily as we continue to struggle to accept our mortality. But once you have experienced the sense of aliveness that it can bring, choosing acceptance becomes much easier and your life much richer.

Our thoughts form our beliefs which directly affect our emotions and how we feel. It's completely understandable that a diagnosis of cancer can send our thoughts spiralling into worst-case scenarios and exaggerated fearful thoughts that are stressful. But it is important to remember that fear increases the stress hormones, cortisol and epinephrine, in our body (the so-called fight-or-flight hormones). This increase can in turn lead to cellular inflammation which encourages cancer cells to grow (see Chapter 10). In her book *Conscious Medicine*, Gill Edwards explains how stress actually slows down the healing process and in some cases can make disease prevention and healing impossible as the immune system is not able to work effectively when the body is in fight-or-flight response.

So making the emotional shift to acceptance, thereby reducing internal stress is an incredibly important principle in maintaining and improving overall health. In her book *Loving What Is*, Byron Katie describes how she came to discover a very powerful tool called 'The Work' (see Resources

Section). The author leads us through a structured process of examining our thoughts and helps us to accept the reality of the situation rather than lament or get angry at what is or what isn't.

Research has shown that while living with cancer, it makes sense to eat well, take gentle exercise, and use meditation and other techniques to enable you to have moments of relaxation and above all be gentle on yourself. Throughout our journeys we have found a number of alternative simple self-help and complementary therapies to be beneficial and have described some of them in Chapters 6 & 7.

Use the Cancer Card!

- Don't be afraid to use the cancer card every now and then.

- Don't waste your time doing things you don't want to do. If you've been invited to a party that's sure to bore the pants off you – don't go!

- If someone starts dumping their emotional baggage onto you, pull the card and run for the nearest exit – you don't need this!

- But be careful not to overuse it and remember just because you have cancer it doesn't mean you can get away with bad behaviour so choose your words and your actions wisely!

- Use cancer as an opportunity to put yourself first.

Part 2
Listen To Your Body and Take Control

The Cancer Journey

CHAPTER 6
Self-Help Techniques

Visualisation

Ongoing research has shown that visualisation (also known as guided imagery) can improve the emotional wellbeing of people with cancer. It also has a positive physiological effect.

A group of women with breast cancer, who practiced relaxation and visualisation techniques, produced noticeable psychological and immunological improvements, (e.g. higher white blood cells which play a central role in immunity and kill tumour cells). Relaxation training in acute non-surgical cancer therapy has been shown to be highly effective in reducing symptoms such as nausea, discomfort and blood pressure, while improving emotional measures such as anxiety, depression and fatigue (see Reference Section).

Given the positive results that visualisation produces, its simplicity to practice and its ability to enhance our overall mood, we believe it is essential to our wellbeing and encourage you to try it.

Visualisation is a mental exercise that uses the imagination to create a desired goal. It is something we do both consciously and unconsciously. Take someone who is a worrier and always imagines the worst. They are creating a negative internal representation of their world, and by visualising a negative outcome they are performing a form of mental programming leading to a pessimistic view of life. The power of thought is very real. Thought is energy and we can learn to mobilise this energy towards enhancing our quality of life. By adopting a positive outlook, envisioning a good outcome and focusing on pleasurable thoughts we create a natural state of happiness and well being.

In his book *How the Mind Can Heal Your Body*, Dr David Hamilton explains that 'the brain doesn't seem to know the difference between real and imaginary, which serves our purpose if we want to visualize ourselves recovering from an illness'. He goes on to list numerous case studies where people have dramatically improved their health using visualisation. But how can we make use of this information now and what practical benefits can be gained from it?

We can take advantage of this by using our brain to promote health and well-being by just imagining it. It sounds too simple to be true but when you consider that every single function our body carries out, it does so because our brain tells it to. By just thinking about it, this gives us the power to become healthier. Neuroscience studies have now conclusively shown that if we think about moving a part of the body, the area of the brain that governs that movement, is stimulated. Hamilton says 'Several recent studies have shown that stroke patients and people with spinal cord damage could regain some movement by imagining themselves moving.'

So we can use visualisation to imagine a vibrant healthy body, beaming with vitality from the inside out, rather than dwelling on the cancer cells taking over our body. Believing that you have a healthy body, while making necessary lifestyle changes, goes a very long way to feeling and becoming healthier. Remember that thoughts become things, so choose to be positive and visualise health over thinking negatively and focusing on disease.

Author and visualisation authority Shakti Gawain says 'Creative visualisation – as it is also known – is the technique of using your imagination to create what you want in your life', claiming the power of visualisation is only limited by our imagination.

This idea is based on the premise that everything begins with a thought, then either consciously or unconsciously we use our imagination to fuel it. This will either create something that nurtures us or limits us – so choose your imaginings wisely.

Visualisation has proved popular with the psychology community and the results are extremely useful for those of us with cancer. This evidence can be used to encourage us to use visualisation in ways specific to our situation. Psychologists have also shown that visualisation can be a powerful tool in improving sporting ability. The classic experiment often cited is how three groups of students were chosen at random, with no experience of visualisation. The first group practiced playing basketball daily for 20 days. The second group abstained from practice altogether and the third group spent twenty minutes each day for the 20 days visualising themselves playing basket ball and successfully scoring by throwing the ball into the net.

After twenty days the group that had actually practiced improved 24%. The second group didn't improve at all. But the third group who had only visualised improved an incredible 23%. This is exceptionally good news for those of us suffering from fatigue or illness. It shows visualisation can influence our brain to send messages to our muscles resulting in muscular micro movements. This may help with keeping some degree of muscle tone and reinforce the neural pathways for movement.

For some of us, particularly when we are very fatigued or unwell, it is not possible to exercise, and at times like these it can be helpful to try visualisation. If you are too tired to attend that yoga class or haven't got the energy to go for a walk, visualising is a great alternative. There are several ways to do this.

One simple technique to try would be to begin by sitting upright if this is comfortable, using cushions for support if necessary. You may prefer to lie down but it is harder to stay awake in this position. Close your eyes and take several deep breaths and then imagine a giant movie screen and watch yourself doing the yoga class, noticing how you perform the postures. See yourself as fit and healthy – this is you as you would like yourself to be. Above all notice that you have a smile on your face and allow yourself to enjoy the freedom of movement you are displaying on the screen. Then imagine you can step into the 'you' on the movie screen and are able to perform the way 'the revitalised healthy you' was doing.

The same applies to visualising walking in nature. See yourself with an upright posture, moving freely, breathing easily and smiling. Imagine yourself either in the forest or strolling along the beach and picture the scene as clearly as possible in your mind – the colours of objects surrounding you, the feel of your feet on the leafy forest floor or in the warm sand. Be completely aware of what's happening around you. Make the image in your mind as bright and as detailed as possible, even imagine the smells and the feel of the air on your skin as you walk.

If the movie screen technique seems a little complicated, you may find it easier to just imagine yourself actually being in the yoga class or going for the walk. Imagine you are performing the movements and be aware of everything about the environment around you. Listening to a Yoga CD and burning incense can be helpful as can listening to a CD with either woodland or ocean sounds.

The key to successful visualisation is to bring in as many of your senses as possible – hearing, smell, taste, sight and touch.

We feel it might be helpful to talk about the many uses and claims made regarding visualisation. As there are three authors writing this book it is only natural that we have different views on its uses. However, what we are all agreed on is that visualisation is a useful tool to help us combat stress, and it is proven to be beneficial in combating muscle wasting as well as enhancing a sense of well being. You will undoubtedly hear of people visualising battle scenes between the body's natural defences and the cancer cells. The drawback with this kind of imagery is that it can stimulate the fight or flight response in our bodies, increasing adrenalin secretion, and enhancing the primary stress reaction. We prefer a more gentle approach such as relaxing and imagining the body being filled with a healing golden light.

> Thoughts become things (this book started as a thought!) so be sure to maintain a positive outlook as it can make all the difference.

Meditation

Meditation is just taking deep relaxation one stage further, and there are probably as many ways to meditate as there are teachers of the technique! In general, though, meditation draws our awareness to our inner stillness and allows us to experience a deep sense of calm and restorative peace. Learning and practising the art of meditation can help us tolerate the emotional reactions and anxieties of life threatening disease. Our brains are constantly growing, something scientists call 'neural plasticity'. As we think and use the muscles in our brain, millions of brain cells connect with each other creating a 'brain map' for each function our body carries out. The brain is like a muscle which gets stronger the more it is used. So if you are used to complaining a lot, you will have built up brain maps to support your negative thoughts and emotions. However if you were to decide that you are going to be positive and practise positive affirmations and gratitude, your brain map associated with positivity will grow, while the negative map gets smaller, resulting in you becoming a naturally happier and more positive person. David Hamilton describes how meditation increases the prefrontal-cortex of the brain – the area of the brain that controls concentration, free will and compassion. When we connect with love and compassion, it releases natural feel-good hormones such as dopamine into our body which makes us feel good, lowers blood pressure, and slows ageing. It also reduces inflammation, the type of environment which cancer thrives in.

The following practices will help you to cope more effectively. When you meditate, find a comfortable position to sit – either on the floor or in a chair. Don't lie down as this may cause you to drift off to sleep rather than meditate.

Mantra meditation:
This first meditation is based on a mantra; it is the repetition of a chosen word such as Peace or Calm. It can be any word that invokes a sense of stillness or even spirituality for you.

Close your eyes and begin to notice the whole of your body. Are you comfortable or do you need to make any changes to how you're sitting? Start by following your breathing and listening to the sound of your breath. There is no need to change it just observe it. After a few moments begin to repeat your chosen word, repeating it as you inhale and again as you exhale. As thoughts enter your mind, gently notice them and return to the word, carrying on repeating it in time with your breathing. If you lose your focus and find yourself thinking 'Oh, I forgot to hang the washing out' or 'I must call Linda', simply start over again repeating the word as you inhale and exhale. Do this for twenty minutes then stop repeating the word. Sit for a few moments then slowly open your eyes. You will be pleasantly surprised at the difference this meditation can make to your day.

Flame meditation:
This form of meditation uses the power of fire to dissolve negativity.

Put a candle on a table and sit so you can look directly into the flame, not down on it. Silently focus on the flame. Send any negative thoughts to the flame and allow them to dissolve and burn away. Try not to pay any attention to their content; just sacrifice them into the flame. In your mind's eye see your mind emptying of all negativity and filling with pure loving light, inner peace and tranquillity. After about five minutes slowly close your eyes and take your thoughts back to the rest of your body and the sounds in the room. Move a little, stretch your muscles and gently re-open your eyes and blow out the candle.

During meditation our minds are still alert to our surroundings and we can easily step back into the here and now any time if the need arises.

Mindfulness meditation:

'Mindfulness – It means paying attention in a particular way – on purpose, in the present moment and non-judgementally.' Jon Kabat-Zinn (scientist, writer, meditation teacher and founder of The Stress Clinic at the University of Massachusetts Medical Centre).

We spend so much time thinking about yesterday and worrying about our future that we often forget about the here and now. What we must try to remember is our power is always in the present moment. The past is gone, we can't be sure of the future, all we have is now. If you remember that you always have a choice in every moment, every moment becomes a choice. Whatever happens, happens. It's how you choose to react to it that matters. Buddhist monk, teacher, author and peace activist, Thich Nhat Hanh says 'Life can be found only in the present moment. The past is gone, the future is not yet here, and if we do not go back to ourselves in the present moment, we cannot be in touch with life.'

An exercise for you to try:

Find somewhere quiet and comfortable. Sit on a chair, or the floor, keeping your spine upright if possible – you might need some cushions for support. The idea is to be able to sit and stay awake but be comfortable. Some people find it helpful to imagine a golden thread attached to the top of their head gently pulling them upwards so they are able to sit with the head, neck and spine in alignment.

As you sit in this comfortable position, spend a few moments noticing the different sensations in your body. Then turn your attention to your thoughts, notice the constant cycle of thinking, planning and remembering. There is no need to try to change them – all you need to do is notice them. Turning your attention to your breathing; feel the air moving in and out of your body. Gradually become aware of the sensations of air in your nostrils. Is it cooler as you inhale and warmer as you exhale? Be aware as thoughts come into your mind. There is no need to try and change them, just notice them and become aware of how easy it is to get drawn into the cycle of thinking, remembering and planning. As this happens, keep returning to the breath inhaling and exhaling, using your breathing as an anchor. Do this for as long as you wish.

When you come to the end of your mediation sit for a minute or two before getting up, giving yourself time to come back into your surroundings.

Loving-kindness meditation:

One of the things that can happen when we are caught in the grip of a serious illness or a very difficult time, is that we shut down and turn off our feelings. By closing the doors to our heart we hope to become like little hedgehogs with a prickly exterior that protects us on the outside and keep us safe on the inside. It seems as though our instincts drive us into shut down so we can preserve the energy needed for our bodies to engage in the healing process. You may have noticed when you're feeling unwell that you just want to curl up under the duvet and sleep. Often the last thing you want is company or, God forbid, intimacy. Yet one thing we need constantly throughout our illness is love. We can imagine you're all groaning now we've mentioned the four-letter word but we believe it's true. Research shows that humans appear to function better when there is some kind of expression of love in their lives. While this can be in the form of loving support from caring friends and family or loving affection from partners, it can also be from a pet such as a dog. Research has shown people who have lost a partner respond much better when owning a pet that brings 'loving' affection into their lives.

When we shut-down, the positive intention is to take care of ourselves, but shutting down for a long period of time is not always the most beneficial way of looking after ourselves. The result can be that we isolate ourselves, becoming withdrawn and uncommunicative and this can be detrimental to our well-being.

Is there any way of using our need to withdraw without alienating ourselves from the people who love and care for us? There are steps we can take by putting together a few simple practices that can gently transform our lives. One exercise known as 'Loving Kindness' is wonderful for generating a sense of wellbeing toward yourself and others.

Although it is easy to do, it can unleash a tsunami of emotions and feelings. These reactions can vary from feeling yourself filled with loving acceptance to feelings of sadness and anger as stored up tensions are released. With this exercise you are gradually eased out of shutdown.

To practice loving kindness allow about 20 minutes for this exercise. First find a quiet place where you are unlikely to be disturbed, sit down and make yourself comfortable closing your eyes and gently turning your attention to your breathing. Just observe your breathing, and as you begin to settle down begin to say to yourself the following:

> *May I be well.*
> *May I be filled with loving-kindness.*
> *May I be peaceful and at ease.*
> *May I be happy.*

Keep repeating the phrases over and over again and you will gradually begin to sense feelings of peace, happiness and loving kindness.

Practising for twenty minutes each day can gradually bring us out of shutdown and open our hearts to embrace life and love ourselves.

Walking in Nature as Meditation:

Walking is another form of meditation as it gives us a break from all the stresses and strains we are surrounded by at home. Until you are able to have some peace free from mobile phones, TV and laptops, only then do you realise how much calmer you feel! Walking in nature allows us the time and space to reconnect with the world and with nature. You'll find yourself smiling at the butterfly landing on a leaf and listen to the birds singing their wonderful unique sounds. You will start to feel calmer, lighter and appreciative of the beautiful scenes that we take for granted when we are moving at 100 miles per hour. This can reduce stress which, as we've mentioned earlier, depletes the immune system and the body's ability to fight disease. So take a walk on the wild side!

Exercise

You may consider taking up a gentle exercise regime such as yoga or QiGong. These forms of exercise work primarily to unite body, mind and soul, and are, in their own way, another form of meditation that allow your body's energy to feel balanced and rejuvenated. There are many forms of yoga so do some research until you find something that resonates with you. When you practice regularly, progression and improved flexibility comes quickly.

Caution – some exercises may not be suitable, for example arm movements after surgery in the armpit and jogging for patients with bone metastases. It is always sensible to consult your consultant/oncologist before undertaking any physical activities.

However, if you feel too tired, fatigued or simply would rather stick pins in your eyes than do anything more physical than breathing, then listen to your body! It is vital you give your body the rest it needs. One of the things we feel very strongly about is to do whatever is right for you. Give yourself permission to be the best judge of what is best for you both physically and emotionally at any given moment in time.

> A breath of fresh air can help to revitalise your body and mind.

If you do feel you might benefit from going for a gentle walk but are either not motivated to go by yourself or even nervous if you're not feeling very strong, this might be the ideal time to involve someone else. We often find that friends want to help but it's sometimes difficult to think of anything constructive they can do. Getting out in the fresh air and walking with a friend is such a pleasurable thing to do. It is good for you, and friends are usually delighted to be asked! If you do decide to walk on your own make sure to take a charged mobile phone with you, and establish in advance if you can get public transport or some other means of getting home in case you feel unwell or too tired to carry on.

Exercise visualisation can be another helpful alternative (see Visualisation section earlier in this chapter).

Breathing

Breathing exercises can be very useful to combat the effects of anxiety. Unlike other visceral bodily functions such as digestion or circulation, breathing is the only totally autonomous function which we can easily regulate by the conscious mind. Breathing exercises can be done by anyone and virtually at any place and time, and as well as helping to reduce anxiety it can be both restorative and energising.

At times it can seem impossible to find rest and relaxation with our minds going round and round in circles. One deceptively simple but extremely effective breathing exercise that has many benefits including generating a sense of calm and improved sleep, is known as alternate nostril breathing. This technique has a harmonising effect between the right and left sides of the brain, bringing with it a sense of calm.

Alternate Nostril Breathing Exercise:

Step one: Close your right nostril by gently pressing your right thumb against it then exhale through the left nostril.

Step two: Inhale through the left nostril, then close your left nostril using your fingers on the same hand.

Pause for a moment.

Step three: Open the right nostril by moving the thumb and exhale through the right nostril.

Step four: Inhale through the right nostril starting cycle all over again.

Pause for a moment.

Sit quietly for a few moments after you have finished.

This simple exercise is so easy to do but complicated to write down. Here is a condensed form of the technique:

> BREATHE in through the left nostril,
> PAUSE.
> Breathe out through the right nostril,
> Breathe in through the right,
> PAUSE.
> Breathe out through the left nostril,
> Breathe in through the left,
> PAUSE.

Here's another example of a very **Simple Controlled Breathing Exercise**: Sit comfortably, close your eyes and become aware of your breathing. Follow it in and out. Don't consciously alter your rhythm just follow the breath as it naturally flows in and out. Inevitably after a few minutes your mind will become distracted and drawn to other thoughts. The essential art of the exercise is to gently acknowledge these thoughts, push them to the side and bring your attention fully back to your breathing. Do this whenever you can and for as long as you wish.

There are lots of different types of breathing and deep breathing exercises which are useful in helping to achieve a relaxed state of mind. They can also be valuable in helping you fall asleep.

Mindfulness – Be In The Here And Now

Another useful exercise to get into the habit of doing is checking in with yourself. Doing this for two or three minutes a day can be very beneficial. It can be done standing or sitting – the beauty of standing is you can do it while waiting for a bus or in the supermarket queue. You may close your eyes if your environment allows and you're not prone to dizziness. First notice your posture, how you are standing or sitting, are you feeling any tension in your body? There is no need to do anything about it, just acknowledge it. Then take a few deep breaths and ask yourself, 'How am I feeling at this moment?' Notice your reply and then let it go. There is no need to dwell on it. Once again notice your posture. Are your feet flat on the floor? Are you sitting straight or hunched? Perhaps make some slight adjustments or not. Now come back to your breathing allowing your thoughts to pass through your mind like soft clouds in a summer sky. No need to change them or pursue them just let them go. Then ask once again how you are feeling, then let it go and open your eyes if you had closed them.

Bottling up emotions is a very natural reaction but there can be great value in finding a way to release them, especially if you can do this in your own time and space. It may seem odd to suggest you'll ever need anything else to help you cry after a cancer diagnosis but you might be surprised at how you can suppress your sadness.

Just in case you need a boost to get all the tears out of the way, here are some movie suggestions to help open the flood gates.

10 Films to Make You Cry

The Notebook
Eternal Sunshine of the Spotless Mind
Green Mile
Beaches
Romeo and Juliet
Titanic
The Neverending Story
Ghost
Jack & Sarah
Saving Private Ryan

Sleep

We're all aware of the importance of sleep to our physical health and emotional well-being. And, as fatigue is a common side-effect of cancer and cancer treatment, it's important to allow yourself as much sleep as you feel you need. Your body is designed to heal and repair itself through the course of the night, so it's vital you get 8 hours of quality sleep, ideally between the hours of 10pm and 6am. Snacking before bed, and eating your dinner too late, can disrupt the body's ability to effectively carry out its job as the energy that would normally be used for healing is diverted elsewhere to help digest the food. So to avoid this, try to finish eating your last meal at least three hours before you hit the sack.

If you have trouble sleeping due to anxiety, cancer paranoia (where you fear every lump and bump is more cancer) or stress, try listening to a relaxation CD or practising meditation just before bed to help calm your mind. (Also see the section on insomnia in Chapter 3.)

Here's an exercise for you to try when you need help going to sleep: Lay on your right hand side, close your right nostril with your right hand and breathe entirely through your left nostril. Repeat for 10 inhalations. This will access the right hemisphere of your brain bringing about a calming effect.

Your quality of sleep can also be affected by your surroundings so make sure you turn off all electrical appliances in your bedroom, including your mobile phone or even better, remove them completely to make it into a peaceful comforting boudoir! Absorbing electro-smog while you sleep is not conducive to healing your body. Also try to sleep in complete darkness as any leakage of light into the room you're sleeping in plays havoc with the pineal gland and will greatly reduce how rested you feel on waking.

CHAPTER 7

Pamper Your Body & Soul

– Holistic/Complementary Therapies

Reflexology – Put Your Best Foot Forward!

In the past 10 years or so, reflexology has become one of the most popular alternative therapies used by those suffering from cancer. It is a complementary and holistic treatment, which involves applying pressure to a specific area, or 'reflex' on either the hands or feet. According to reflexologists, these areas match every part of your body; there is a map of the left side of your body on your left foot, and the right side of your body on your right foot. For example, an area in the ball of your left foot represents your left lung and your right big toe represents the right side of your head.

Although there is no scientific evidence to prove that reflexology can cure or prevent any type of disease including cancer, it has been shown to help with cancer symptoms such as pain, nausea and anxiety. Reflexology massage works by stimulating energy pathways in the reflex areas (similar to those used in acupuncture – see below). This can improve circulation and encourage the body's natural healing process and restore energy and balance. The many other benefits include promoting a deep feeling of relaxation, reducing stress, anxiety and help with digestion problems such as constipation.

Massage – Soothe Operator

Massage therapy is a treatment that works to relax you mentally and physically. The therapist uses a variety of techniques including stroking, tapping, pressing or kneading the soft tissues of the body and these can range from being soft and gentle to vigorous and brisk. Massage therapy has been shown to offer many benefits to people coping with cancer and these include better sleep patterns, improved psychological wellbeing and less anxiety and depression. The main reason for this has been shown to be associated with increased levels of the mood-regulating chemicals serotonin and dopamine which are released by the body during massage.

Aromatherapy Massage – Scents and Sensibilities

Aromatherapy means therapy 'using smell'. Aromatherapy combines the physical and emotional effects of gentle massage with the medical and psychotherapeutic properties of essential oils. There are dozens of different essential oils and these are extracted from various flowers, plants, fruits, resins, barks or roots and distilled to produce a pure essence. All of them have different characteristics and therapeutic properties. The therapist adds the oils to the massage medium and as the scents are inhaled the smell travels up into the part of our brain called the limbic system. When stimulated, this area of the brain releases feel-good chemicals such as endorphins and other neurotransmitters which can make us feel relaxed, calmed and can even reduce sensations of pain. Based on which benefits we need most e.g., de-stressed, energised etc, the therapist will select the appropriate essential oils or combination of oils which are likely to have the best therapeutic effect.

Acupuncture – No Pins Just Needles & No Pain Just Gain!

Acupuncture has been used with significant success on people with various problems. Although there is no evidence to show that it can treat or cure any illness, it has been demonstrated to help relieve cancer pain and also some of the symptoms and side effects associated with cancer treatment.

It is a holistic complementary therapy with its roots in ancient Chinese medicine. The traditional technique involves inserting very fine disposable stainless steel needles through the skin at specific points on the body (acupoints). Other well known acupuncture methods include acupressure where the therapist uses their fingers to apply pressure to the acupoints and electroacupunture in which a weak electrical current is sent through the acupuncture needles into the acupoints. The acupuncture practitioner will determine which acupoints relate to the problem being treated and will then insert the needles into the appropriate part of the body. They may move or twirl them at different depths or speeds and/or heat or electrically charge them, or in the case of acupressure, massage the appropriate acupoints.

Following treatment with acupuncture, people report feeling relaxed and with an improved sense of well being. Those with specific medical problems have also experienced relief from pain and discomfort, reduction in a number of side effects including chemotherapy-induced nausea and vomiting, dry mouth, sleep disorders, cancer-related tiredness, hot flushes and night sweats and chemotherapy-induced peripheral neuropathy (nerve damage causing numbness, tingling, change in sensation).

So if you're suffering from any of the above, a visit to an acupuncturist might be just the solution. And even if you just feel more rested and relaxed after your treatment it would be worth a try.

Reiki – The Vessel of Calm

Reiki is the Japanese method of using 'Universal Energy' to enhance well-being. The word Reiki is made up of two Japanese words – Rei which means 'God's Wisdom or the Higher Power' and Ki which is 'life force energy'. So Reiki is actually 'spiritually guided life force energy'. Universal energy flows through all of us – however this can become blocked during stress and illness.

The technique involves a gentle 'laying on of hands' to remove blockages and restore the flow of energy, which is thought to bring peace and balance to the mind, body and spirit.

Although Reiki is a hands-on form of healing, unlike some other therapies, no manipulation or removal of clothes is involved. It is likely you will lie down on a bed and be asked to close your eyes. You may feel the practitioner's hands resting gently on a part of your body while directing the energy to you, although some may not make contact, simply choosing to hover their hands above you instead. The healing is believed to direct itself naturally to where it is most needed in the body with the Reiki practitioner acting merely as a conduit, through which the Universal energy is drawn into the receiver. At the end of the session, you should feel a sense of calm, balance and relaxation.

While the greatest benefits of Reiki is relaxation it can also relieve headaches and general pain, reduce blood pressure and improve sleep patterns. Reiki has also been shown to be a powerful aid in helping recovery following surgery and chemotherapy in people with cancer.

Coaching – Give Yourself Your Life Back!

Another holistic therapy which can be useful to those of us dealing with cancer is life coaching. Once we come to terms with our diagnosis many of us feel an overwhelming desire to make the most of the rest of our lives. But it's sometimes really difficult to know how to turn this determination into specific changes and also to be sure these changes are what we truly want. A coach can help you identify what is really important to you, what would give you the most joy and satisfaction and increase your chances of fulfilling your dreams. Coaching can help you identify goals and make the changes necessary by giving you practical tools, step-by-step guidance, support and the motivation to succeed. Identifying what you need and setting goals to achieve this can energise and empower you to transition from feeling helpless because of your diagnosis, to being back in control and feeling confident. A coach can provide us with inspiration, courage, focus and determination to create our best life now!

> 'Time is free, but it's priceless. You can't own it, but you can use it. You can't keep it, but you can spend it. Once you've lost it, you can never get it back.'
> *Harvey MacKay (business book author, speaker & columnist).*

Coaching exercise:

A coaching session will usually start with the coach asking you lots of questions, and here are a few of the types of questions they might pose to you. Try answering the following;

1. **What in your life gives you most joy?**

   A few examples might be your children, spending time with your family and friends, listening to music, reading a great book, walking with nature, having a massage, getting/giving a hug.

2. What challenge or goal could you set to achieve more of one or all of these things in your life?

3. If you were well/healthier/had more energy, what would you be doing now that you're not doing?

4. What is your greatest fear?

What would you do differently if you knew this would definitely happen?

What would you do differently if you knew this would definitely not happen?

5. What barriers exist that you feel prevent you from achieving your goals or dreams?

6. How can you overcome these and who could help you?

7. What steps are you willing to take to achieve your goal(s)?

8. When are you going to start?

Case study:

Matilda was feeling very low having just received a diagnosis of secondary cancer. She was retired and lived on her own but had very strong support from her family and her church. She had been extremely positive and had fought hard through her first cancer journey and had had a clean bill of health for almost 10 years, but felt now that she didn't have either the energy or motivation to go through it all again.

With her coach Pam, she looked at the areas of her life which she felt discouraged by and they identified that one of her biggest fears was of being on her own. During her first diagnosis and treatment she had a pet dog and said that when she was at home she never felt alone. The dog had unfortunately died a couple of years ago and she had not replaced it. Although she dearly missed the company, especially now that she was facing this horrible ordeal, it was unthinkable for her to get another pet at this moment in her life.

Matilda told Pam that while she had access to the many various pets of her family and friends, nothing compared to the feeling of 'not being alone' that having her dog in the house had given her, particularly at night. The coach suggested she share her concerns with her loved ones which she agreed to do. (Often just talking to friends about your worries and fears can enable them to feel involved and be supportive by allowing you to off-load and can therefore be beneficial to both parties.)

The solution which came out of this was that one of Matilda's nieces was about to start university. This niece had a pet parrot and it was decided that the parrot should move in with Auntie Matilda! The parrot was a very chatty African Grey male who adored company but was very low maintenance. Family and friends were only too happy to volunteer to look after the parrot as and when Matilda was in hospital or didn't feel well enough, and someone would always come to clean out the cage for her. Within a few weeks of having the parrot Matilda said she felt emotionally much stronger and ready to deal with the ordeal of her treatment regime, and she loved the company of her feathered companion. Both she and the parrot had also learned some new vocabulary!

Often a coach can help you address your fears in a way that family, friends and even your doctors can't do. They will help you look for and find what is holding you back or frightening you, and together, you can identify a way forward and open yourself to a new world of opportunities (see Resources Section).

CHAPTER 8

Express Yourself – Live Life, Be Brave, Find the New You!

It is important during a stressful or traumatic period of your life to stay connected to yourself and your feelings. Self-expression is about communicating your feelings by 'doing'. Being able to achieve something through our own efforts and creativity gives us a sense of purpose and boosts our self confidence, inner strength and optimism. Any form of expression is helpful whether it's finger-painting, creative baking, photography or taking up trampolining (providing you are up to it physically of course!). We have listed some suggestions for things that we have tried and found to be both enjoyable and therapeutic.

Keeping a Journal

This has been scientifically proven by Dr James W Pennebaker, psychologist at the University of Texas, not only to be good for our emotional health but also our physical health. His book *Opening Up* is filled with information on why suppressing inner problems takes a devastating toll on health; how long-buried trauma affects the immune system and how writing about your problems can improve your health. In Chapter 5 we talked about the benefits of keeping a gratitude journal and also suggested that writing an anger journal can also be a useful exercise. For others, just regularly writing about anything and everything, putting their thoughts and feelings into words, can be surprisingly therapeutic. Particularly if you are holding onto powerful emotions without really expressing them, journaling about them can be a great way of releasing this internal stress. And you don't need to have any regard for the usual rules of writing such as spelling, grammar or logical sequence as it's for your eyes only!

'There is a vitality, a life force, an energy, a quickening that translates through you into action, and because there is only one of you in all time, this expression is unique. And if you block it, it will never exist through any other medium and will be lost.'
Martha Graham (leading modern dance and choreography pioneer).

In her book, *The Artist's Way*, Julia Cameron recommends her students and readers write what she calls, 'Morning pages' every day to help release their blocked creativity. This involves writing three A4-sized pages of longhand writing without editing or judging what comes out. It is 'strictly stream-of-consciousness' she says. It might look something like this: 'Oh I can't be bothered to do this. Did I get my dry-cleaning yesterday? I don't have anything to say, I'm so tired, I must go food shopping!' The idea behind this is to get all the whiny, petty, negative stuff out on the page so it's not clogging up your mind and, therefore, gives you an outlet for all your frustrations, without having to carry them around with you. This is obviously similar to keeping a journal only you write every little last thought as and when it comes and as its purpose is just to clear your mind, it's not necessary for you to read back through. It merely helps in what Cameron calls 'brain-draining'. We recommend it as a way of processing your feelings about your cancer.

Writing

Since our cancer diagnoses, all three of us have turned to writing as a form of self-expression and therapy. This has been in the format of our websites with regular blogging and also the book that you currently have in your hands. But it's absolutely not necessary to intend publishing to benefit from the therapeutic effects of writing. It can be in the format of poetry, short stories, letters, your inner ideas and dreams, or even your autobiography! Anything which gets your creative juices flowing will give you a sense of purpose and personal achievement.

Cooking

Getting your hands dirty in the kitchen could be a great way to express your creativity by giving your brain a rest and your creative self the chance to concoct some fabulous healthy meals for you, your friends or your family. By participating in an activity which is creativity-led or by doing something monotonous, where the body instinctively knows what to do without having to consciously apply it; such as driving, rollerskating, cycling or cooking, we are able to rest the left hand side of our brain and activate our more creative right brain. This kind of activity promotes health and wellbeing by helping us to relax as well as allowing us to sub-consciously process our thoughts and emotions.

Gardening

Gardening is known to promote both physical and mental health. We're not sure exactly why, but there seems to be an innate attraction between people, plants and nature, and being outdoors creates feelings of tranquillity, appreciation and peace. Even if your energy levels are very low or you're feeling unwell, being out in the fresh air and in touch with nature can restore and lift the spirits. Research has shown that just spending time in nature lowers stress hormones, reduces blood pressure and boosts endorphins – the body's feel-good chemicals. Whether it's a single window box, a little plot or a large garden; growing something as simple as one tomato plant can give you a sense of joy, purpose and achievement. Family and friends will often be happy to become involved and help, and a joint project can bring shared joy and pleasure.

> Getting back to nature

If the physical side of gardening is not for you, a great way of getting the benefits of being in touch with nature is to feed the garden birds. You can hang up one or two simple bird feeders or erect a bird table and, as water is just as important as food, installing a bird bath is also a lovely idea and a joy to watch being used. By providing year-round supplies of food and water, we can actually help make a difference to the local bird population and to bird conservation. One of our friends who enjoys feeding and watching the birds in her garden went one stage further. During her cancer treatment she decided to keep her hair as it fell out. A few months later when the breeding season started, she put little clumps of her hair out amongst the branches of the trees in her garden for the birds to use for nest-making. She reported that they seemed to love it and she enjoyed watching them busily flitting around collecting it. A very novel and rewarding way of re-cycling!

If you don't have a garden, perhaps you could visit your local park or pond and feed the wildlife there. You'll be doing your bit for nature and benefiting yourself in return.

So with all these positive benefits of tending your garden and its creatures, isn't it time you got outside?

Music Therapy

Music has been shown to affect specific areas of the brain, and music therapy is known to have a positive effect on emotional well-being. Reports suggest that jazz is one of the best genres to lift the spirits!

It doesn't seem to matter whether we play, sing or just listen to music it can improve our sense of self-awareness and boost feelings of relaxation. Studies in people having chemotherapy have reported that listening to music during treatment can reduce perceptions of the levels of pain and nausea.

Climb every mountain!

Having realised that time was not as unlimited as previously thought, Pam decided to pursue a lifetime's ambition of learning to play the piano. Despite a very gentle and patient teacher, progress was stifled by an almost total lack of musical ability! However, she can testify to the fact that the focus required is a good distraction and a great way to de-stress.

Another friend with cancer has taken up singing lessons and says she finds it both calming and energising. The social interaction with others has also provided a boost to her self-esteem. Her progress is happily much better than Pam's so it's unlikely they will ever form a duet! So why not consider looking into some form of music therapy or perhaps listen to your favourite music at times of stress?

Art Therapy

Art therapy is a way of expressing specific emotional or physical issues through art. It's not about creating a wonderful piece of art – in fact you don't even need to be able to draw or paint – it's about creating a visual representation of your inner-most thoughts and feelings. It can offer a safe way to express difficult, sensitive or destructive emotions through being creative rather than talking, and embraces the idea that the process of making art is therapeutic. As with many types of complementary therapies, art therapy can be useful for people coping with cancer and can help them explore otherwise suppressed emotions such as fear, depression, anger or grief.

It has been shown in cancer patients to reduce a broad range of symptoms related to anxiety and pain. People using art as a healing therapy have reported feeling more in control and in touch with their inner thoughts and this in turn has empowered them. They also report having fun in the process. While many people choose to express themselves without analysing their creations, an art therapist can help an individual interpret their art in order to reveal the meaning in their creations.

The Cancer Journey

CHAPTER 9

What Family and Friends Can Do To Help

When a cancer diagnosis rocks your world, it affects not only you but everyone around you. Whether they are family members, friends or colleagues, concerns for your wellbeing ripple through your community and affects everyone in different ways. Family and friends, often themselves reeling from the shock of the diagnosis, may want to assist you but may not have the first clue of what they can do to help.

So, we have listed below some things which we've found useful and other ideas that we wish the people around us had thought of.

Tips on How to Communicate with a Cancer Survivor

- Never use the word 'victim' when speaking to or about someone with cancer. They are 'living with cancer', 'a cancer survivor' or even doing just fine'!

- Be aware of your body language. There's nothing more annoying than someone's face with 'poor you' plastered all over it. Obviously we want to know you care but be careful not to pity us or patronise us.

- If you write to us, be as positive as possible and make it clear that you don't expect a reply to your letter or email.

- We mentioned earlier about sending round robin emails to update friends and non-immediate family and you could offer to set up email groups.

- When you're visiting try to keep conversations light and have humour high on the agenda – laughter really is the best medicine.

- We don't always mean what we say. Everything can be very confusing so please don't question us too much or take anything as set in stone.

Please allow us to be grumpy and angry but don't be overly sympathetic.

- Be aware that how we feel just now could be radically different to how we feel tomorrow or even in a few hours from now.

Useful Things That Can Be Done By Family And Friends

- Your initial reaction may be to send flowers or a plant which is a lovely gesture, but please send them already in a vase/container so that they don't need any work.

- Being a good listener is definitely the best thing you can do. But try also to be intuitive as sometimes we'll want to talk and other times we won't.

- Bringing a meal which can be easily heated up and served will usually be very well received but do check first about dietary requirements. Homemade soup is usually something that is welcome especially if our appetite is poor.

- Volunteer to do some housework such as cleaning or laundry. Check areas like the kitchen and bathroom where it's easy for dirt to build up but would take a lot of effort for someone ill to clean and cause angst if we notice it's dirty. With laundry, if feasible take it away and bring it back done or, if this isn't possible, do it in the house but try to be subtle so that we don't feel guilty!

- Do some gardening. Planting something pretty to look forward to next season will always be appreciated.

- Send us some lovely organic chemical-free beauty products so we can pamper ourselves in the comfort of our own home.

- If there are children involved there are lots of things which would be helpful eg. school run, playing with them (colouring, board games, taking them out of the house either to the park, for a walk or even a special treat). A sick parent will often feel very guilty that the children are suffering as they are not able to give them as much attention as they would like. Also be a good listener/sounding board for them and let them know they can talk to you. Often children don't want to ask their parents difficult questions for fear of causing upset and they might find it easier to talk to someone else.

- If we're well enough to go out you could bring a little fun into our lives by taking us on a shopping trip, or to the cinema, or out for a drive in the countryside. If we want to stay at home you could bring a video to watch with us (see below) or do a foot and leg massage and maybe a pedicure.

- A subscription to a favourite magazine always makes a lovely gift – especially if we're housebound.

- Offer to stay with the patient to give the partner/carer a break. As the patient we know the constant stress our carers/partners are under (Pam has also experienced being in this role). Giving our carer a special treat such as a relaxing therapy session like a massage or similar would probably be very well received. Equally, just being able to go out for a couple of hours knowing we've got uplifting company, would be valuable.

- Arrange a relaxing treat for the patient if you think they'd appreciate it. Be careful to select a registered therapist and speak to them in advance so that they fully understand that a) the client has cancer and b) they are accepting and supportive of a last minute cancellation. And if possible pick a therapist who you feel will be sensitive and uplifting rather than overly sombre. You could look into whether they do home visits as this could be helpful to those of us unable or unwilling to leave the house.

- Plan treats ahead to give something to look forward to such as a concert or the theatre but again be sensitive that things may need to be cancelled at the last minute.

- Christmas can be a particularly difficult time and offering to help with getting presents either by going shopping or helping to internet shop may be helpful.

- Offer to walk and feed animals.

- If you know that we want it and you feel capable of doing this, it can be helpful to offer to carry out some internet research into our type of cancer. There is an overwhelming amount of information available, lots of which may be inaccurate, frightening or morbid so it will need to be filtered.

Laughter is often the best medicine!

10 Films to Make You Laugh

There's Something About Mary

Wedding Crashers

The Hangover

Yes Man

Meet The Parents

The 40 Year Old Virgin

American Pie

Dumb and Dumber

Life of Brian

Blazing Saddles

We've also put together a list of things which we either found to be at best annoying and at worst upsetting.

- Don't say I wish there was something I could do. If you genuinely want to help there's lots you can do!

- Don't talk to us in hushed tones and don't cry around us. Other peoples' fears and tears are hard work.

- If you offer help and it's declined please don't take offence. Being respectful of our wishes is much more helpful than trying to cajole us.

- Please don't voice your concerns about our treatments, unless we ask for your opinion and/or advice, and be supportive of our choices even if you've got reservations.

- Don't tell us stories of other people's cancer. We don't want to hear about old Betty Horne from down the lane who died of cancer – this is neither helpful nor uplifting for us!

- Don't tell us how to think or feel. Being told to think positively rarely has the desired effect.

- Being a good listener is really important but please understand that there may be times when we really don't want to talk so don't try to push us into it.

- There's a difference between 'How are you?' to 'How ARE you?' One's just a general, how you doing; like you would say to any 'healthy' person but the latter is a deeper more meaningful question that is looking for a deep heartfelt answer as to how we REALLY feel. We don't always want to describe how we really feel so let us bring it up, rather than you.

- Don't make us feel guilty about not being in touch. Please don't leave us voicemails or emails asking us to call so you won't worry – we will call in our own time!

If you are the partner it's very easy to forget about your own needs but it's really important that you look after your own health and wellbeing. Please try to accept as much help and support as you can.

Very often the patient will put a brave face on things for visitors, especially if they are trying to be positive and boost spirits. But sometimes, after the guests have left the family or carer is left to pick up the pieces as the patient plummets both physically and mentally. If you are the carer, please be selective with the visitors you do allow and let them know if you think they might cause the patient to deteriorate, and suggest that they just stay a few minutes or perhaps do something for the patient which doesn't involve them talking or appearing brave, such as a gentle hand or foot massage while having relaxing music in the background.

Part 3
Living and Eating Consciously

The Cancer Journey

CHAPTER 10

Eating Consciously

Nature and Nurture

We have all heard the old adage, 'You are what you eat,' but how often do we really think about what we are putting into our bodies? With our busy lives, we often grab food on the go as it's quick and easy, but this often means we end up filling up on heavily processed snacks without thinking about what fuel we are giving our bodies to run on. For our body to work effectively, we must nourish it with real food abundant with vitamins, minerals, enzymes and phytonutrients.

In this section we will look at the different ways you can support your body whether you are at the beginning of your cancer journey, slap bang in the middle of having treatment or through the other side. There are many ways to improve your current health using food as your medicine. It is important however, to understand the 'why's' behind changing your diet. This will empower you and enable you to make better food choices in the future. First let's look at what really makes cancer tick.

> 'You are what you eat. You are what you think.'
> *Louise Hay*

How Cancer Thinks

Cancer cells possess abnormal genes which instruct them to continue multiplying, ignoring signals from surrounding tissues to stop. They then secrete a poison to these tissues which creates a local inflammation. From there, the cancer cells send messages to nearby blood vessels causing new blood vessels to grow towards them, effectively hi-jacking the blood supply for its own use, eventually resulting in a tumour. This process is called **angiogenesis.**

In his book *Anticancer: A New Way Of Life,* leading physician, neuroscientist and author, Dr David Servan-Schreiber outlines the circumstances where these cells are encouraged not to carry out this process:

1. When the immune system works against them.

2. When the body denies the cancer cells the **inflammatory environment** they need to grow.

3. When blood vessels refuse to reproduce the environment the cancer cells need to flourish.

It's important to know that some foods have an anti-inflammatory effect on the body and some have pro-inflammatory effects and we will look at both of these in this chapter. So, by carefully choosing what we put into and onto our body, we can reinforce the above mechanisms that prevent the disease from taking hold. If cancer is already present, we can use this knowledge to adapt our diet and lifestyle alongside conventional treatment to give our bodies the best possible chance of mobilizing against the disease.

Cancer Cell Suicide

As well as making our bodies as inhospitable to cancer cells as possible, by changing our dietary habits and preventing angiogenesis, we can promote **apoptosis**. Apoptosis is when the cancer cell decides to end its life and actually self-destructs. This is of course something we definitely want to encourage!

One of the ways to do this is by choosing food and drink that contain polyphenols known as catechins. One of these, EGCG (epigallocatechin gallate) is found in green tea and is one of the most powerful molecules against the growth of cancer.

In his book *Anticancer – A New Way Of Life*, Dr Servan-Schreiber explains 'All in all, by stimulating our immune cells, fighting inflammation (with nutrition, physical exercise and emotional balance), and fighting angiogenesis, we undercut cancer's spread. Acting in parallel with strictly conventional medical approaches, we can enhance our body's' resources.'

Now that we understand cancer and its weaknesses, we can look at what our body needs to work optimally and what changes we can make to our lifestyle and diet to promote this.

Acid versus Alkaline

Different organs within the body require different pH environments. The pH scale is used for measuring how acid or alkaline something is. To give you some idea, the acidity scale ranges from 0-6.9 and the alkalinity scale from 7 – 14, with 7.365 being the optimal pH for our blood. Slightly on the alkaline side is where we should aim for our pH level to be, and this can be achieved by eating a balanced diet rich in alkalizing oxygen-rich foods. There are some parts of the body, however, that prefer a slightly acidic environment such as the stomach, colon and bladder.

By choosing an anti-inflammatory (which as we learnt earlier prevents cancer cell growth) alkaline, low glycaemic diet full of whole foods, we provide our body with an optimum environment in which to create health. In contrast, an acidic environment creates the potential for our body to develop anything from a cold to chronic fatigue to cancer. So it is really important to make the connection between the food you are eating and the effect it has on your body – to eat consciously.

When the body is too acidic, the lymph system, liver and kidneys all become overworked trying to remove the acidosis from the body. This also puts our immune system under great stress which, if faced with an illness, is certainly not an additional problem we want to deal with. Acidity is caused by consuming too many highly acidic foods such as meat, dairy products, alcohol, white refined sugar and simple carbohydrates. We need some acidity in our diet but not as much as the average person is consuming through a Standard UK diet (appropriately abbreviated to SUK!).

> Highly acidic foods promote inflammation which promotes cancer cell growth.

On the following page we have put together a list of some alkaline and acidic foods to help you choose what to eat and how often;

There are several types of acidic food and drink that feature heavily in the average person's diet and although we recommend eliminating as many of them as possible, we realise this might be a big adjustment. So, to make it easier for you, we have split these foods into three groups:

1. acidic foods that should be avoided at all costs; these foods are highly addictive, highly acidic, mucous-forming, allergenic and pro-inflammatory.

2. acidic foods that are highly acidic that should be consumed very occasionally if at all; these foods are highly addictive, highly acidic and pro-inflammatory but can be consumed **on occasion** should you wish to continue to do so.

3. acidic foods that offer nutritional benefits and should be consumed in moderation as part of a healthy diet.

> If the thought of completely eliminating any of the above foods is daunting, we would suggest you begin by gradually reducing your intake of them as they are detrimental to your body's natural pH balance, overworking your liver and creating a toxic inner environment.

1. Highly Acidic Foods – Avoid	2. Highly Acidic Foods – Consume very occasionally	3. Acidic Foods – Consume in moderation
Dairy products: milk, cheese, butter	Alcohol	Dried fruit[3]: apricot, currant, cranberry, raisin
Fizzy Drinks	Animal protein: red meat, poultry, fish, eggs	Fruit; cooked tomato, cranberry, plum
Highly refined foods: white sugar, white bread, white pasta, flour, rice, wheat	Drinks: Black tea, coffee, decaffeinated coffee	Grains and legumes: chick pea, black bean, kidney bean, oat
Nuts: roasted and salted nuts and all peanuts[1]		Nuts[4]: hazelnut, macadamia, pecan, pine nut, walnut
Highly refined oils: soybean, sunflower, corn, hydrogenated (trans) fats, margarine		Processed soy products[5]
Soya milk[2]		Sweeteners: honey, agave syrup (also known as agave nectar), raw honey, yacon syrup
Sweeteners: brown sugar, corn syrup, dextrose, fructose, maple syrup[2]		
Table salt		
Vinegar		

1 Conventional and organically harvested peanuts contain a type of mould that produces a toxin called aflatoxin which is carcinogenic (cancer-causing). Additionally, non-organic and even organic peanuts are heavily treated with pesticides.

2 See Reading Between the Lines (next section).

3 Buy un-sulphured dried fruits where possible to avoid consuming any harmful sulphur dioxide which acts as a preservative and can be an allergen for some people.

4 Nuts are packed full of healthy fats, enzymes, vitamins and minerals but some are more acidic than others which is why they fall into the moderation pile. They should be consumed as part of a balanced (mostly) plant-based diet.

5 Raw soy beans contain a type of mould that produces a poisonous toxin called aflatoxin. This is only removed during the fermentation process making soy, tempeh, miso and tamari safe for consumption. Westernised soy is processed and not fermented meaning that the carcinogenic aflatoxin remains intact.

Alkaline Foods – Consume generously

Apple cider vinegar

Cold-pressed oils: olive, argan, borage, coconut, hemp, flax

Coconut water and coconut butter

Cultured and fermented foods: raw sauerkraut, kimchi, kefir

Green leaves: kale, lettuce, cabbage, spinach, collard greens, watercress, rocket, endive

Fruits: avocado, lemon, lime

Herbs: parsley, rosemary, mint, coriander, basil etc

Nuts: almond, brazil

Seeds: flax, hemp, sesame, chia, sunflower

Sea vegetables: arame, dulse, hijiki, kelp, nori, wakame, kombu

Sprouts: alfalfa, broccoli, mung bean, lentil, quinoa, radish, sunflower etc

Vegetables: asparagus, aubergine, broccoli, Brussels sprouts, cabbage, cauliflower, celery, courgette, fennel, green beans, leeks, onions, peas, raw tomato, etc

Root vegetables: beetroot, carrot, sweet potato, turnip

The foods listed above all vary in their acidity and alkalinity; some are more alkaline or acidic than others. We are not suggesting that you remove all acidic foods from your diet as the body does require some degree of acidity. However, we recommend you eliminate the foods that are highly acidic while incorporating more alkalising foods into your diet to keep your pH level within a healthy range. By cutting out the bad stuff and adding in more of the good stuff, you'll be giving your body a helping hand to work effectively.

Please note this list is not exhaustive and we recommend you use the information provided in the Resources Section of this book to research alkaline foods further.

If you are considering reducing or eliminating animal products from your diet, you might be wondering where you would get your protein from. Well, thanks to some very clever advertising, we have been led to believe that we need more protein than we actually do. In fact, in Dr T. Colin Campbell's 2006 book, The China Study, his research shows that as protein consumption increases, so do the rates of chronic disease. This is because most of our protein intake comes from animal products that are high in saturated fat which promote yes, you guessed it, inflammation. According to www.dietaryfood.com, we only need approximately 46 grams of protein per day and this can easily be achieved through eating a varied vegetarian plant-based diet with foods such as almonds, broccoli, buckwheat, cashew nuts, flaxseeds, hemp seeds, kale, lentils, quinoa, spinach, sweet potato, spirulina and chlorella, to name a few!

Reading Between The Lines

Unfortunately there is an over-abundance of foods that contain additives such as artificial sweeteners, colourings, flavour enhancers such as MSG, hydrogenated fats and many more which are often disguised by other names. For example here are just some of the other names sneaky manufacturers use to disguise sugar:

- **Brown sugar**
- **Corn syrup**
- **Dextrose**
- **Fructose**
- **Fruit juice concentrate**
- **Glucose**
- **High-fructose corn syrup**
- **Honey**
- **Invert sugar**
- **Lactose**
- **Maltose**
- **Maple sugar**
- **Molasses**
- **Sucrose**
- **Turbinado**

> Sugar is sugar no matter what name it's assigned, so given that sugar promotes inflammation, try to avoid it where possible and be aware of it lurking in packaged foods.

Dextrose is another name for high-fructose corn syrup and is found in a lot of packaged and processed foods. As processed foods are highly acidic, contain hidden ingredients and promote cancer cell growth, we suggest these foods are eliminated from your diet – altogether forever! When considering what to eat, try to choose fresh ingredients that haven't been tinkered with; that way you can be sure that your body is getting the best fuel possible.

Glycaemic Index

The Glycaemic Index (GI) measures the effect of your food on your blood glucose (blood sugar) level. Foods that are high on the scale tend to have a negative impact on the body and can promote cancer cell growth.

Foods with a high glycaemic index break down quickly sending the amount of glucose in our blood soaring. This puts the body under pressure to regain a healthy level. If you've ever experienced a sudden burst of energy shortly followed by a slump in energy, it is likely that you consumed one or more high GI foods. Chocolate, breads, sugary snacks and treats are the main culprits. These are all known as 'simple' carbohydrates as they are highly refined and lacking in fibre. Fibre slows down the release of sugar and has a much healthier effect on the body. A carbohydrate with fibre is also known as a 'complex' carbohydrate meaning that it is in its whole form, takes longer to digest and keeps your energy levels stable. It is much better for your body and energy levels to eat low GI foods which release glucose gradually into the bloodstream, keeping your blood glucose level much more stable resulting in continuous slow-releasing energy. Here are a few examples of complex and simple carbs to help you make better food choices;

'Unrefined', 'Good' Complex Carbs	'Refined', 'Bad' Simple Carbs
Whole grains and legumes: adzuki, chickpea, lentil, mung, black-eye pea	White flour, pasta, sugar, bread
Vegetables: green leafy vegetables, root vegetables, salad vegetables, sea vegetables	Biscuits, cookies, cakes, muffins, crisps
	Energy drinks, concentrated fruit juice
	Fizzy drinks
	Fruit*

*Although fruit is a simple carbohydrate, because it contains fibre, it is considered a healthy carb that offers nutritional benefit.

In order to bring our blood glucose level down to a healthy level, the body must release insulin to enable the glucose to enter cells. Our cells use glucose for fuel but if the cell has all it needs, any excess glucose is then stored as fat. This process is also accompanied by the release of a molecule called IGF-1 (Insulin-like Growth Factor) whose role is to stimulate cell growth. By this process the sugar encourages tissues to grow faster promoting inflammation, which as we learnt in the last section, stimulates angiogenesis (cancer cell growth).

Foods and their Glycaemic Index (per gram of carbohydrate)

Low Glycaemic Foods	Medium Glycaemic Foods	High Glycaemic Foods
Bread: sourdough, rye, mixed grains, Essene (otherwise known as Ezekiel, sprouted wheat bread or Manna bread)	Fruit: cantaloupe melon, cherries, papaya, pineapple, raisin	Biscuits, cookies, cakes, muffins, crisps, white flour, pasta, sugar, bread, white pasta, bagels, croissants, muffins,
Fruit: apple, pear, dried apricot, banana, blueberries, grapefruit, grapes, kiwi fruit, mango, orange, peach, pear, strawberries	Wild rice	Fruit: watermelon
Grains: buckwheat, bulgur, quinoa, brown rice		Drinks: artificial sweetened cordials, fizzy drinks, alcohol
Drinks: Green tea, herbal tea		Grains: millet, jasmine rice, white rice, white bread, whole wheat bread, cereals
Root vegetables: sweet potato		Potato: baked, mashed, boiled
Natural sweeteners: stevia, xylitol, agave syrup, yacon syrup		White sugar, brown sugar, honey, maple syrup, fructose, corn syrup,

GI values taken from The New Glucose Revolution by Jennie Brand-Miller and Kaye Foster-Powell. Please note this list is not exhaustive and we recommend you check our Resources Section for books with more information.

So, in short, we must try to avoid eating high glycaemic foods to ensure we do not provide the cancer with the environment it needs to grow. Instead we should adopt a low GI (stable blood sugar), alkaline (optimum for blood pH) diet to give our bodies the best possible environment to create health. We have provided below a brief outline of foods and their glycaemic index to give you an idea of which foods will raise your blood sugar and which will keep it stable.

Be conscious that some foods will vary as to which end of the scale they sit. For example: a food may have a medium GI and therefore be considered okay to eat generously but it might only be one point away from being categorized as high GI, so do bear this in mind.

By consuming a diet of mainly low GI foods, you help to keep your energy stable without spiking your blood sugar or causing inflammation. Many plant foods such as lettuce, kale, broccoli, spinach, celery and cucumber are 0 on the GI Index scale giving another compelling reason to transition towards a diet including these nutrient-packed foods.

> High GI Foods = Insulin release = Inflammation = Cancer Cell Growth

Choosing to Eat Consciously

What we mean by eating consciously is examining our daily diet and the foods that we are eating. If you can, why not do whatever possible to starve those wayward cancer cells? It's sometimes hard to remember that we don't have to be solely at the mercy of doctors and drugs. We can take back some control by exerting our power of choice in what we eat and how we live our lives. This will support our bodies in creating as much health as possible giving us the best chance to fight illness.

Now that we understand how cancer cells operate and what they thrive on, it gives us the knowledge to consciously eat to destroy them, rather than giving them the fertilizer they need to grow.

You can start today by making small changes to your diet by eliminating the highly acidic foods and introducing more alkalising nourishing greens. Should you wish to make more radical changes, it would be wise to consult a qualified nutritionist or health coach to ensure your body and immune system is fully supported. We encourage you to see your food differently – not just something or anything to fill the hunger but a nourishing life-enhancing substance that can dramatically affect the way your body works improving how you look and feel.

Animal Products

As outlined earlier in this chapter animal products, particularly meat and dairy products, should be eaten in moderation if at all. There are several reasons for this. Apart from being highly acidic, they have an extremely negative impact on the body.

According to the National Cancer Institute, cooking meat to high temperatures creates dangerous substances called heterocyclic amines (HCA's) which are carcinogenic and have been known to cause stomach, breast, pancreatic and colon cancer. That alone is reason enough to eliminate animal protein from your diet but additionally, the quality of meat these days is far inferior to that of yesteryear. In an attempt to keep up with supply and demand across the globe, unfortunately our animals are often factory farmed and fed with grains or grass that may have been sprayed with insecticides, fungicides and pesticides. They may have also been reared in a stressful and possibly less than ideal environment. Also, due to their lack of exercise they often become lame or unwell and are consequently pumped full of antibiotics to treat infection and disease. When we eat these animals, we absorb all of these elements which add to our body's toxic load putting it under unnecessary additional stress.

'80-90% of all cancers, cardiovascular diseases, and other degenerative illness can be prevented, at least until very old age, simply by adopting a plant-based diet.'

Dr. T Colin Campbell, author of *The China Study: The Most Comprehensive Study of Nutrition Ever Conducted and the Startling Implications for Diet, Weight Loss and Long-term Health*

Due to the lactose contained within cow's milk many people experience problems digesting dairy products. This can cause inflammation, bloating, allergies, eczema and asthma. Lactose is also used in some chocolate, biscuits and breakfast cereals. In his book *The China Study: The Most Comprehensive Study of Nutrition Ever Conducted and the Startling Implications for Diet, Weight Loss and Long-term Health,* Dr Campbell explains that a protein called casein, which makes up 87 percent of cow's milk, promotes cancer cell growth. So we can see a very clear and scary link between meat, dairy products and cancer, giving us one more reason to reduce or eliminate where possible.

Protein can also be sourced by eating fish, however be aware of what type of fish you are consuming and where it comes from. Like intensively-reared cows and pigs, farmed fish often develop illnesses and disease. Also be aware that the bigger the fish you eat, the higher it will be in the food chain and therefore more likely to contain harmful chemicals and pollutants that are unfortunately found in our oceans.

If you do feel you would like to keep animal products in your diet, we would suggest you buy organic produce in order to reduce the volume of toxins your body and immune system are subjected to.

More Natural Raw Food

By now you will hopefully understand that an anti-inflammatory, low GI, alkaline plant-based diet will stack the health odds in your favour. If the idea of a plant-based diet seems scary or confusing, let us explain. But first we want to fill you in on the power of chlorophyll.

Go Green

Chlorophyll is the green substance in plants that allows them to absorb light from the sun and convert it into usable energy. It is often referred to as the blood of the plant. When we eat or drink foods high in chlorophyll such as kale, broccoli, spinach and chard for example, we send light and oxygen to every cell in our body. Chlorophyll helps the body to build red blood cells, boost the immune system and reduce inflammation while promoting healthy cell activity. Chlorophyll has also been shown to produce an unfavourable environment for bacterial growth in the body and, therefore, helps to fight free radicals, effectively increasing the body's resistance to illness. So you can see why it is so important to eat a diet high in gorgeous greens!

Wheatgrass, which contains extremely high levels of chlorophyll, is considered to be a complete food in itself. It contains many amino acids, enzymes, minerals and vitamins that help to detoxify the liver and bloodstream, while protecting us from cancer-causing agents. It has also been used to successfully treat many gastrointestinal tract illnesses as well as constipation and diarrhoea. It is thought that just one pound of fresh wheatgrass juice is equivalent in nutritional value to 23 pounds of garden vegetables.

Enzymes Equal Energy

Enzymes are required for nearly every single bodily function. Although the body has its own natural reserve of enzymes which are essential for digestion and good health, as we get older, our body's natural production of enzymes becomes less efficient and it relies on us to replenish the reserve through the food we eat. The problem is that enzymes are heat-sensitive meaning they get completely destroyed when heated above 118°F (46°C). So when we eat cooked food, our body is forced to use the enzymes from its own stock in order to digest the food we are eating. If we continue to do this without replenishing the supply through eating nutrient-dense, enzyme-rich foods which are available only in raw uncooked foods, our enzyme reserve becomes severely depleted and leaves our body lacking in important building blocks for everyday cellular activity.

As well as all of the enzymes being lost by cooking, it is also thought that up to 70% of the vitamins and some of the minerals also get destroyed when exposed to high temperatures. So although we may be eating a healthy diet full of cooked vegetables, we may find that we aren't getting as many nutrients as we think. We are not suggesting that you eat only raw food, but by increasing the amount of raw food you consume, you considerably reduce the energy your body has to exert for digestion and helps the body with many other functions.

Question – So what can I eat?
Answer – Fresh, natural, whole foods

When faced with any illness, we can support our body's immune system by giving it as much pure unadulterated natural rocket fuel in the form of raw goodness as possible. Even just a green juice or green smoothie will go a long way to filling you with much-needed nutrients to help boost your immunity (see recipes in Chapter 11 for ideas).

We can't stress enough how important it is to really understand that your illness is hugely affected by the things you put into and onto your body. We have been blessed with a wonderful machine that keeps us running all day every day, even when we are unconscious and tucked up in bed. But eventually it will begin to let us down if we neglect and don't help it!

The exciting thing about introducing more raw food into your diet is that quick and tasty meals can be made and eaten straight away! From delicious 'pasta' dishes to scrumptious blueberry pie! Please see our Recipe section for inspiration in Chapter 11.

Essential Fatty Acids

Omega-3 and Omega-6 are otherwise known as essential fatty acids and they are called 'essential' because the human body cannot make them. So we must ensure we obtain what we need from the foods we eat. For optimum health, the body needs a perfectly balanced ratio of omega-3 and omega-6.

What are they good for?

Omega-3's play a vital role in brain function as well as helping to develop the nervous system, reduce inflammation and the proliferation of inflammatory diseases such as cancer, arthritis and heart disease. Omega-3's are found in green vegetables, flaxseeds, pumpkin seeds, walnuts, nori, hemp seeds, fish, organic grass-fed meat products and some dairy products (although we would recommend you consume the majority from non-animal sources for the reasons outlined earlier in this section). In addition, it is also important to understand that products from animals that are reared intensively and fed corn, soy or wheat instead of grass, contain almost no omega-3. They do however contain omega-6 which our bodies do need, but in moderate amounts and in proportion to our intake of omega-3. It is very easy to consume too much omega-6, especially if we are eating a standard Westernised diet as most packaged and fast food products have been cooked in, or contain an over-abundance of hydrogenated oils that are high in omega-6. When our intake of omega-3 and omega-6 becomes unbalanced, we increase the inflammation in our body which encourages cancer cell growth and inflammatory-related illnesses such as arthritis, diabetes and Crohn's disease, to name a few.

Omega -6's are responsible for storing fats and play a crucial role in healthy growth and development. When consumed in the right balance with omega-3, it also plays a role in *reduction* of inflammation in the body. Like omega-3, omega-6 is essential and it can help with osteoporosis, ADHD, arthritis and cancer but as explained above we must be careful not to consume excessive amounts and we must ensure the quality that we are eating is obtained from whole natural foods, as opposed to harmful processed foods and oils.

The best way to ensure you consume a healthy ratio is to increase the amount from whole food sources such as flaxseeds, flax oil, hemp seeds, hemp oil, chia seeds and green vegetables while reducing the intake of harmful heated vegetable oils such as sunflower, canola and corn. Additionally cut down or eliminate foods containing hydrogenated fats such as processed and packaged foods that have an ingredient list as long as your arm and a shelf life deeming it edible for your grandchildren when they're 50! Okay, we're exaggerating but you get the gist.

You may recoil at the idea of eating seeds but a small bowl on your desk or kitchen top will remind you to graze on them throughout the day, keeping your energy up with nutritious foods designed to nourish you from the inside out.

You may feel uncomfortable at the thought of eating new foods and changing the way you eat, but if you want to improve your health and be an active participant in your wellbeing, then you may need to open your mind to new knowledge as with it comes empowerment.

> 'Clearly, in every country there is a direct connection between the cancer rate and the consumption of meat, cold cuts and milk products. Conversely, the richer a country's diet in vegetables and legumes (peas, beans, lentils), the lower the cancer rate.'
> Dr David Servan-Schreiber, *Anti-Cancer – A New Way of Life.*

Superfoods

What IS a superfood? Well, superfood is the term commonly used to describe a food with a high phytonutrient content that may bestow health benefits. **Phytonutrient** is the term given to naturally occurring plant compounds which are thought to help reduce inflammation, strengthen the immune system and protect against cancer.

Three words are mentioned frequently in the following section so to save you having to flick back to previous pages, here's a little reminder:

Angiogenesis: the process in which cancer cells hi-jack surrounding blood vessels to support their growth.

Inflammation: the environment in which cancer cells thrive.

Apoptosis: when the cancer cell decides to end its life (cancer cell suicide).

We have listed a few 'superfoods' rich in phytonutrients below, but instead of regarding them as special foods, these are just foods that should be the foundation of our everyday diet. We will introduce you to **real** superfoods in a minute.

Berries
Strawberries, blueberries, raspberries and blackberries contain phytochemicals which protect the body from free radicals.

Citrus fruit
Lemons, limes, oranges, tangerines and their peel are said to possess anti-inflammatory flavenoids and help to detoxify the liver. Grapefruit is also included in this list although there are contradictory reports on whether it should be consumed while undergoing cancer treatment.

Cruciferous vegetables
Kale, broccoli, cabbage, cauliflower, collard greens, bok choy are thought to contain cancer-fighting properties.

Garlic
Garlic has antiviral, antibacterial and antifungal properties.

Ginger
Ginger helps to reduce inflammation and is a powerful antioxidant.

Green tea
Green tea is rich is polyphenols thought to promote apoptosis and prevent angiogenesis.

Goji berries
Goji berries are packed with cancer-fighting beta-carotene, amino acids, Vitamin B, B2, B6 and Vitamin C.

Herbs
Herbs are purported to contain specific healing properties and promote apoptosis; parsley is rich in chlorophyll making it a powerful cleanser and detoxifier as well as anti-inflammatory; coriander aids digestion and helps cure diarrhoea; rosemary contains powerful antioxidants and anti-inflammatory properties.

Matcha
Matcha is a green tea powder that contains 137 times the antioxidants of regular green tea.

Mushroom
Shiitake, maiitake, enoki, crimini, oyster and portabello mushrooms contain lentinans and polysaccharides which help boost immunity.

Pomegranate
Pomegranate contains anti-inflammatory properties and is rich in antioxidants.

Sea Vegetables
Sea vegetables are packed full of iodine which help to regulate the thyroid as well as many minerals and trace minerals essential for optimal health. Sources include; nori,dulse, wakame, hijiki, arame and kombu.

Tomatoes
Cooked tomatoes contain lycopene which is thought to protect against cancer. However tomatoes change from an alkaline state to acidic when heated so eat them raw whenever possible.

Turmeric

Turmeric promotes apoptosis and is an extremely powerful anti-inflammatory food source.

Watermelon

Watermelon is rich in cancer-fighting lycopene and beta-carotene. Its seeds also offer vitamin E and the mineral zinc.

Wheatgrass

Wheatgrass is a potent source of chlorophyll, enzymes and amino acids which helps to cleanse the blood, increase red-blood count, detoxify the liver and protect us from carcinogens.

Eat Your Sprouts!

Sprouts? Yes sprouts! But we're not talking about good old Brussels, although they are very good for you. The sprouts we are talking about are what you get when you soak nuts, seeds, grains and legumes. The process of sprouting activates germination which increases their enzyme and nutrient content. It is thought that broccoli sprouts contain as much as 50 times the cancer-fighting compound than mature broccoli! By consuming more sprouted foods we help to replenish our body's natural enzyme reserve, while giving our body a rest from the energy-zapping job of digestion.

How do I Sprout?

It's pretty simple really. All you have to do is soak the nut, seed or grain that you want to sprout, pop them in a glass bowl, jar, nut milk bag, clean pop sock or sprouting tray, rinse and drain approximately twice a day and watch them grow. Sprouting trays are available to buy online as are seeds such as alfalfa and broccoli which are some of the most nutritious sprouts you can eat. Soaking and harvesting times do vary so we would suggest you check the Resources Section for sprouting books that we recommend. There is also a vast amount of information on sprouting available on the internet.

What Can I Sprout?

You can sprout anything from alfalfa to almonds, from barley to buckwheat, from sesame seeds to spelt. The result will differ depending on what you are sprouting. For example, just by soaking almonds in water for approximately 8 hours or more they will swell, removing the enzyme inhibitor therefore activating and increasing the enzyme content. After soaking, they should be drained and rinsed and used within 3 days. Keep stored in the refrigerator until ready for consumption.

Mung beans, lentils, chick peas, radish and quinoa sprouts will begin to grow little tails anywhere between 1 and 4 days and are easily sprouted in a bowl or jar. Alfalfa and broccoli seeds like to grow for approximately 5 days until they are about 3cm long and standing tall so we find a sprouting tray is best to grow them in. It's important to rinse them through at least twice a day. Chick peas and buckwheat prefer to be rinsed more often so be prepared to keep an eye on them.

Make them a feature of your windowsill or breakfast area so you remember to look after them and eat them. Just a few teaspoons of seeds will yield pounds of nutritious sprouts making them easy on the wallet.

Healthy Helpers

Now you know the types of foods that should be making the foundation of your diet, here are some additional ways to enhance your nutritional intake. Please note that these are not in any way designed to replace food but merely a way to augment your health levels.

Omega-3 and Omega-6

Udo's Oil is an organic nutritionally superior, fish-and gluten-free source of essential fatty acids which are crucial for healthy cell structure and brain function.

Vitamin D

Vitamin D has anti-inflammatory effects and has been shown to considerably reduce the risk of several types of cancer and heart disease. It also plays an important role in supporting the immune system and creating strong bones. Make sure you get outside for twenty minutes a day for your Vitamin D fix!

Selenium

Selenium helps to stimulate immune cells and can be found in Brazil nuts and organically grown vegetables. (Unfortunately non-organic produce does not possess this mineral as the intensive harvesting process strips the farmland of all selenium content.)

Probiotics

Between 70-80% of the body's immune system lives in our digestive tract. The body requires a delicate balance of both "good" and "bad" intestinal bacteria which if left unchecked, can cause anything from gas to bloating to indigestion to Candida which can spiral into more serious degenerative diseases. Our "good" bacteria can easily get wiped out by an overly acidic diet as well as drugs such as antibiotics and chemotherapy. By taking good quality probiotics you help to maintain and restore a healthy balance of bacteria.

Fermented foods

Another fantastic way to restore gut harmony is by eating naturally fermented foods such as raw sauerkraut, kimchi and kefir. These foods contain high levels of good bacteria as well as B vitamins. Other fermented foods beneficial for health include organic apple cider vinegar, unpasteurised miso, unpasteurised tamari (wheat-free, gluten-free soy sauce) and nutritional yeast.

Digestive Enzymes

As we've discussed, a healthy digestive system is crucial for optimum health. By adding digestive enzymes to your diet, you lessen the amount of work your body must do in digesting your food. This enables your energy to be redirected elsewhere to repair and heal which is definitely something we want to promote.

Vitamin B12

It is impossible to obtain Vitamin B12 from a vegan plant-based diet as Vitamin B12 is created by microorganisms in soil and water which are then consumed by animals. So if you're thinking of going vegan, then you will definitely need to use supplementation for your B12 fix. A good quality all-round B vitamin supplement will deliver what you need, or if you prefer, you can take only B12 supplements.

Real Superfoods

Açai
Açai is a purple berry that grows in Brazil and contains ten times the antioxidants of grapes and is thought to increase energy levels, improve digestion, increase mental clarity and strengthen the immune system.

Algae
Blue-green algae (BGA) contain extremely high levels of chlorophyll which we know is extremely detoxifying and health-affirming. The two most common BGA's that you may have heard of are Spirulina and Chlorella which are packed full of protein, vitamins and minerals. Spirulina helps to build blood cells, boost immunity, improve concentration and focus, while Chlorella helps to bind and remove heavy metals from the body, counteract side-effects from radiation, reduce inflammation and much more. We could go on and on about this awesome algae.

E3Live
E3Live is a freshwater edible source of blue-green algae rich in vitamins, minerals and phytonutrients and is thought to be one of the world's best superfoods.

Aloe-Vera Juice
Aloe-vera boosts the immune system, is anti-inflammatory, antibacterial and antiviral. Apart from being used to treat sunburn, it is also thought to improve asthma symptoms, help with immunodeficiency diseases and calm ailments such as irritable bowel syndrome (IBS), colitis and ulcers.

Bee Pollen
Bee pollen contains every single known vitamin, twenty-seven minerals and twenty-two amino acids making at a fantastic source of protein. It also contains all of the important B vitamins, including the elusive B12.

Camu Camu

Camu Camu is a Peruvian bush which produces berries thought to be the richest source of Vitamin C known, as well as having anti-viral and immune-boosting properties.

Hemp Protein Powder

Hemp protein powder is high in easily digestible protein and contains the optimal ratio of Omega-3 to Omega-6 essential fatty acids as well as many amino acids and antioxidants. Add to smoothies or sprinkle on salads.

Methylsulfonylmethane (MSM)

MSM crystals are a safe and naturally occurring form of the mineral sulphur which is thought to help strengthen and thicken hair, promote soft skin and strong nails. It helps in the absorption of nutrients and is a natural remedy for inflammatory conditions helping to improve flexibility. Add to drinking water.

Schizandra

The schizandra vine produces berries that have been used in Chinese medicine to treat infections, combat insomnia, boost the immune system and protect the liver. It is also thought to reduce side-effects of chemotherapy and radiotherapy and to improve recovery post-surgery.

There are many real superfoods that offer an abundance of nutrition and have natural properties to boost health. The above foods are just a starting point so we recommend you do some research as there's plenty out there!

See Resources Section for more information.

Juices and Smoothies

Health in a Glass

By now you know that vitamins, minerals, enzymes and phytonutrients are essential for optimum health. But the idea of chowing down of a ton of vegetables to get our vitamin fix isn't exactly appealing, which is why juicing is so fantastic.

Drinking fresh living juice is one of the most health-affirming actions you can take and is an easy way to get access to those much-needed nutrients. Putting fruits and vegetables through a juice extractor simply separates the juice from the fibre leaving you with a glass full of beautiful fresh living juice full of antioxidants. These fight free radicals (otherwise known as oxidants) which contribute to many illnesses including cancer and heart disease. Plus the nutrients contained in fresh juices are utilized by the body far more quickly than those the body obtains from solid food – delivering a stack of nutrients in super fast time.

From his book *The Juice Masters Ultimate Fast Food,* Jason Vale explains that 'In the United Kingdom, one person dies every 3 minutes from coronary heart disease, but research from Cambridge University found that eating one apple a day cuts the risk of premature death from heart disease by 20%, add one orange and one banana and it goes up to 50%. Imagine what 2 pints of live juice would do for you!'

Smoothies are also a fantastic way to drink your greens. The difference between juices and smoothies is that all of the fibre from the fruit or vegetable is used in the smoothie making it a thicker consistency which will leave you feeling fuller for longer. They are packed full of vitamins, minerals and fibre and make a brilliant vehicle for delivering superfoods like blue-green algae, wheatgrass and hemp protein powder to all of your cells. Smoothies take minutes to make and can be easily kept in a drinking bottle or container so you can keep nourished on the go. They make the perfect chemo-buddy!

Household juicers, high-speed blenders, and juice and smoothie recipe books are available in stores and online. Not only are juices and smoothies great for your health but they can help reduce side-effects from cancer-treatment too. Try some of the recipes in the following chapter next time you need something to quell your nausea or calm your headache.

The Cancer Journey

CHAPTER 11

Recipes

Release your inner Nigella or Jamie!

These recipes have been provided so that you can introduce foods into your diet that you may not have previously eaten or considered eating. We would encourage you to try them as they really do taste great and being 'raw', they have the added benefit of giving your body truck loads of enzymes, vitamins and minerals. Remember that by not cooking the fruit, nut or vegetable you will be obtaining the maximum nutritional content available.

Just a quick heads up though before we get started. Some of our recipes mention a dehydrator which is an appliance that is used by a lot of people eating a mainly raw food diet. As nutrients get severely damaged and enzymes completely destroyed in the normal cooking process, those eating a raw food diet do not heat their food over 118° Fahrenheit thus maintaining the foods nutritional content. A dehydrator gently dries food out – as opposed to cooking it – resulting in a crunchier and crispier version of the food that went in, while leaving all the nutrients intact. If you do not own a dehydrator, you can place the food in a fan-assisted oven, keeping it on the lowest setting leaving the door ajar. Remember that high levels of heat will damage the nutrient content of the food so do bear that in mind and do make sure the temperature remains low.

The strength of your food processor or blender will determine how smooth some of the mixtures in the following section turn out, but rest assured any machine will do. You may just need to add a drop of water or two to help the machine out and get the mixture turning.

A word about salt if we may? White table salt is toxic. It is heavily processed, flash-dried at extreme temperatures and put through a refining process which turns the salt purple! As consumers are unlikely to buy purple salt, it is then chemically bleached and many other things added which include glucose, talcum and aluminium silicate, which act as poisons to the body. So we recommend you avoid conventional table salt and use Celtic Sea Salt or Pink Himalayan Salt instead.

Where Does It Come From?

We have already highlighted that it's important to consider what you are putting into your body and also where your food has come from. It's simple – the more toxins you absorb, the more overworked your body becomes. By reducing the number of pollutants and chemicals you put into and onto your body, you help to keep your immune system strong while minimising the body's toxicity levels. Where possible, we would advise you buy organic produce to avoid consuming harmful chemicals that non-organic food may have been sprayed with. Anything you can do to reduce the toxic load on the body will be of benefit.

Unfortunately organic foods do tend to be more expensive so if budget is an issue and you are able, we would recommend you consider growing your own produce. If this is not possible for you, check out a list put together by the Environmental Working Group (EWP) which outlines which foods contain the least and the highest level of pesticides and decide to buy the most heavily sprayed organic. See the Resource section for more information.

Switching your diet to incorporate more raw food can be challenging if it is a radical change for you, so we have given you some easy options to try. We have tried to make the recipes as simple and as easy as possible so we hope you like our suggestions and, of course, feel free to experiment.

If you are interested in finding out more about using specialist ingredients or the benefits of eating more raw food, please see our Resources Section.

Getting Juicy

While whole fruit is full of vitamins, minerals and enzymes, when juiced, it is stripped of its fibre making the natural sugar found within it more easily available. We've already made the connection between sugar and cancer in an earlier chapter, so be mindful that as healthy and loaded with vitamins as a fruit smoothie is, it will cause your blood sugar to spike. This will make your body release insulin which will in turn create inflammation. For this reason we suggest you don't consume too many fruit smoothies although we have provided you with variations to choose from. As you experiment, try to incorporate as many alkalising greens as possible while using just one or two pieces of fruit to sweeten. A green smoothie is the perfect combination – lots of greens and little bit of fruit. In most juices and smoothies we have used low GI fruit such as apples, pears and berries to counter the harsher tasting greens. This will keep the sugar intake to a minimum, while giving you access to the cleansing chlorophyll.

•

Juices

Spineapple

2 handfuls spinach
½ lime
1 cup parsley
½ pineapple

Instructions: Place all ingredients through a juicer and serve immediately.

What is it good for? The bromelain in pineapple helps to reduce **swelling** and parsley **aids digestion** and **cleanses** the body.

Apple Refresher

4 sticks celery
2 apples
½ cucumber
½ lemon, peeled

Instructions: Place all ingredients through a juicer and serve immediately.

What is it good for? This juice is very refreshing. Cucumbers are full of silica which is a mineral found in every organ and cell in your body. Silica is thought to **improve hair strength** while helping **skin to glow** and **nails to grow.**

....

Tip 1: When juicing citrus fruits, cut away the peel being careful to leave as much of the pith on as possible as this is where a lot of the nutrients are contained.

....

Constipation Catapult

1 pear
1 stick celery
1 apple
½ lemon, peeled

Instructions: Place all ingredients through a juicer and serve immediately.

What is it good for? The title says it all!

Blood Booster

1 raw beetroot, peeled
1 stick celery
2 apples
2 cm ginger root, peeled

Instructions: Place all ingredients through a juicer and serve immediately.

What is it good for? Beetroot is an excellent cleansing and blood-boosting vegetable, celery acts as a diuretic and ginger is a natural anti-inflammatory. This will help to rid the body of **excess water** and **bloating.**

....

Tip 2: When a juice recipe calls for ingredients that contain little or no liquid such as ginger, garlic, lemons, limes and herbs, be sure to add them to the juicer first so they get pushed through the machine by the remaining ingredients to gain maximum benefit.

....

Stodge City

I cup tightly-packed spinach
3 carrots
2 sticks celery
I pear

Instructions: Place all ingredients through a juicer and serve immediately.

What is it good for? Think of this one as a thickening agent for **diarrhoea!** Pear also helps dissolve excess mucus and may improve lung congestion and conditions such as **asthma** and **hayfever.**

....

Tip 3: A slightly under-ripe pear is best for juicing whereas a juicy ripe pear tastes best in a smoothie.

....

Carrot Cleanser

3 carrots
I handful watercress
I lime, peeled
I cup broccoli florets
2 apples

Instructions: Place all ingredients through a juicer and serve immediately.

What is it good for? Watercress is a potent **cleanser** and **blood-builder** thanks to its high chlorophyll content and broccoli is known for its **anti-cancer** properties.

Kale Kicker

1 cup kale
2 sticks celery
1 small handful watercress
2 apples

Instructions: Place all ingredients through a juicer and serve immediately.

What is it good for? Kale and watercress are powerful cleansers and can help alleviate **muscle cramps** and **boost immunity.**

Head Soother

1 fennel bulb
2 apples
½ head romaine lettuce
½ cucumber

Instructions: Place all ingredients through a juicer and serve immediately.

What is it good for? Lettuce and fennel contain calcium and magnesium which are antispasmodic; this juice should help to quieten that pounding **headache** or calm **restless legs**.

Carotene Kick

1 apple
4 medium sized carrots
½ red pepper
1 cm ginger root, peeled

Instructions: Place all ingredients through a juicer and serve immediately.

What is it good for? This juice is packed full of antioxidants and **cancer-fighting** beta-carotene.

....

Tip 4: To make the most of your juice, run the juice pulp through the machine a second time as you may find you can get some additional juice. At the end of juicing, pour approximately 50ml of water through the juicer to help any remaining juice reach the spout.

....

Mint Soother

1 small bunch fresh mint leaves
500 ml water

Instructions: Pour boiled water over the leaves and steep for 5 minutes.

What is it good for? Mint can alleviate symptoms of **nausea** and **cramp** so try a mint tea next time you're feeling a bit peaky.

Ginger Aid

1 inch ginger root, peeled
1 cup water

Instructions: Add a chunk of peeled ginger to a cup of hot water and drink. If you prefer not to leave the ginger in the cup, grate the ginger and squeeze its liquid into hot water instead.

What is it good for? Ginger helps to improve **digestion, circulation** and relieves **nausea, bloating** and **inflammation**.

Smoothies

Sweetly Pear

2 pears, cored
1 stalk celery
1 cup spinach
1 cup water
5-9 basil leaves (to taste)
1 teaspoon stevia (optional)

Instructions: Place all ingredients in a high-speed blender until smooth.

What is it good for? Spinach and pears are both very cleansing and help to **support the digestive system, liver and circulatory system.**

....

Tip 5: Stevia is a natural sweetener that has no calorific value and has no effect on the blood sugar making it suitable for everyone, including diabetics. It comes in powder or liquid form and can be used in smoothies, nut milks, raw desserts and more. It is approximately 30 times sweeter than conventional sugar so use sparingly! If you do not have any stevia to hand, use a drop of honey instead but be aware that it is high GI.

....

Mint Mayhem

2 apples, cored
1 ½ cups spinach
1 cup water
1 tablespoon ground cinnamon
8-10 mint leaves (to taste)

Instructions: Place all ingredients in a high-speed blender until smooth.

What is it good for? Spinach is rich in iron, Vitamin C and beta-carotene making it a powerful **blood builder** and **cancer-fighter**. A study published by the US Department of Agriculture reported that cinnamon has shown reductions in lymphoma cancer cells when consumed as a food (Koppikar, et al 2010).

....

Tip 6: Feel free to add in any superfoods outlined in the previous chapter. Add a teaspoon of blue-green algae or hemp protein powder for a nutritional boost.

....

Hemp Heaven

3 cups kale
½ cucumber
3 apples
½ avocado, flesh only
1 tablespoon shelled hemp seeds
stevia (to taste)

Instructions: Place the kale, cucumber and apples through the juicer. Pour the juice into a high-speed blender and combine with the avocado, hemp seeds and stevia until smooth.

What is it good for? Kale is packed full of vitamins and minerals as well as **anti-cancer nutrients**, hemp seeds are loaded with protein and fatty acids essential for health while apples and cucumber **cleanse the body.**

....

Tip 7: If the fruit you bought during your last shopping trip is starting to ripen too quickly, place it in the fridge until you need it as this will slow the ripening process. This also works for avocados, bananas and fleshy fruit.

....

Black Banana

1 cup black grapes
5 romaine lettuce leaves
1 frozen banana
¼ cup water
1 small handful sunflower sprouts
1 teaspoon chlorella

Instructions: Place all ingredients in a high-speed blender until smooth.

What is it good for? Grapes contain resveratrol which is a powerful **antioxidant** shown to have **anti-cancer properties** while chlorella helps to **boost immunity** and **remove toxins** from the body.

....

Tip 8: It's always a good idea to freeze some fruit for those times you fancy something refreshing and don't have the energy to go shopping or have an empty fruit basket. You can reach into the freezer and pull out a bag of frozen blueberries, strawberries, apple, banana, pear or whatever you have to hand. You can then use these to make a frozen dessert or throw in a blender with a splash of water and some greens for a delicious nutritious smoothie. Fortunately nearly any fruit can be frozen without the nutrient content being affected too much.

....

Purple Almond

1 cup almond milk (see page 132)
1 banana
½ pomegranate, seeds only
¼ cup frozen black grapes
1 papaya, de-seeded

Instructions: Place all ingredients in a high-speed blender until smooth.

What is it good for? Papaya is bursting with **cancer-fighting** beta-carotene, enzymes, Vitamin C and fibre, black grapes are extremely **cleansing** and help to **restore an alkaline balance** while pomegranate is packed full of **antioxidants** which has been shown to **prevent prostate cancer cell growth.**

Protein Powerhouse

¼ cup goji berries, soaked for 15 minutes
1 cup water
2 cups spinach
1 cup blueberries
1 teaspoon camu camu
½ teaspoon açaí powder
2 teaspoons bee pollen
1 tablespoon hemp protein powder
1 small handful of sunflower sprouts or snow pea sprouts
2 frozen bananas

Instructions: Drain the goji berries and discard the soak water. Place them in a high-speed blender with the remaining ingredients until smooth.

What is it good for? What isn't it good for?! Blueberries and açaí contain powerful **antioxidants**, goji berries are packed full of **cancer-fighting** beta-carotene, amino acids, and vitamins B and C, camu camu also contains extremely high levels of vitamin C and bee pollen and hemp protein powder are packed full of protein providing the body with the necessary building blocks for health.

Almond Milk

1 cup almonds
3 cups filtered water
Stevia or agave nectar to taste (optional to sweeten)
1 teaspoon alcohol-free vanilla extract or ½ vanilla pod (optional)

Instructions: Combine the nuts and water in a high-speed blender and blend on high until the nuts are completely broken down. Pour into a nut milk bag and strain. If adding a sweetener, place the milk back in the blender and add to taste. If you do not own a nut milk bag, a clean pop sock or stocking will suffice.

Use almond milk with porridge, muesli or add to a smoothie for a creamy delight. (See **Purple Almond**). You can then use the leftover almond pulp for **Berry Blue Pie**. (See Dessert section)

Nuts contain an enzyme inhibitor whose job is to protect the nut and this can sometimes make them difficult to digest. Soaking nuts before using them increases their enzyme content, maximising the nutritional content and makes them easier on our digestive system.

Almond pulp is what is left over after making **Almond Milk.** It will keep in the freezer for up to 3 months so store it in a container and keep frozen if you're unable to use it immediately. This way there is no wastage and you get to make several meals from just a few nuts!

Starters & Snacks

Cucumber Boats with Hemp Smash

1 cucumber
4 avocado
1 ½ teaspoons salt
2 tablespoons lime juice
¼ cup shelled hemp seeds
1 teaspoon ground turmeric

Instructions: Slice the cucumber in half lengthways and scoop out the flesh from the middle of the two halves. (Discard or use in a juice or smoothie.) Place the remaining ingredients in a bowl and use a fork to smash them together until a chunky mixture is formed. Cut the cucumber halves into desired lengths, spoon some of the mixture into each of the 'boats' and serve. Sprinkle with **Spicy Pumpkin Seeds** for an extra crunch factor.

'Peanut Butter' Boats

1-2 little gem lettuces
¼ cup almond butter
1 tablespoon light tahini
¼ cup water
¼ cup sundried tomatoes, soaked for at least 1 hour or more
½ teaspoon salt
½ teaspoon ground turmeric
½ teaspoon stevia (optional)

Instructions: Cut off the hard end of the lettuces and separate the leaves. Wash and dry them and place them on a plate. Drain the sun-dried tomatoes and discard the soak water. Combine them with the remaining ingredients in a high-speed blender until smooth. You may need to scrape down the sides of the blender to ensure it all mixes in. Place a spoonful of the 'peanut butter' on each lettuce leaf and sprinkle with sunflower seeds or **Spicy Pumpkin Seeds.**

Spicy Pumpkin Seeds

3 cups pumpkin seeds, soaked for at least 4 hours
2 tablespoons agave nectar
1 teaspoon ground coriander
½ teaspoon turmeric
½ teaspoon chilli powder
1 tablespoon cumin
½ teaspoon paprika
2 teaspoons onion salt
½ teaspoon garlic salt

Instructions: Drain the pumpkin seeds, rinse them through and place them in a bowl with the remaining ingredients. Mix together, ensuring all the seeds are covered with the spices and agave nectar. If you have a dehydrator, turn the mixture out onto a non-stick dehydrator sheet and dehydrate at 105° Fahrenheit for 8 hours. Flip them over and dry the other side until all seeds are completely dry and crunchy. If using a fan-assisted oven, line a baking tray with baking paper but remember to keep the oven door open and keep an eye on them.

Kale Crisps with Cheese Topping

When nuts are combined with certain ingredients they taste very similar to cheese. In the recipe below, we combine cashew nuts with red pepper and a few other essential ingredients to create a cheesy mixture for our kale crisps. There are many different varieties of kale so use whichever you have available.

6 cups tightly-packed kale
3 tablespoons olive oil
I tablespoon salt

Cheese Topping
I red bell pepper
Juice of ½ lemon
I teaspoon salt
½ teaspoon paprika
I cup cashew nuts
I tablespoon nutritional yeast (optional but does add a delicious cheesy flavour)

Instructions: Strip the kale from its tough centre stem and combine in a bowl with the olive oil and salt. Massage the leaves with your hands until all leaves are covered. Set aside. In a food processor, mix the cheese topping ingredients until it forms a smooth mixture. Drain and discard any excess liquid from the kale and pour over the cheese mixture. Mix the cheese into the kale with your hands until all the leaves are coated with the cheese. Lay the leaves out on a dehydrator sheet and dehydrate for 12-18 hours until crispy.

....

Tip 9: This cheese mixture can also be used as a dip with crudités or served on cucumber boats. (See earlier recipe.)

....

Recipes

Main Courses

Lemon Basil Linguine

2 medium courgettes

Lemon Basil Sauce

½ cup pine nuts
½ cup tightly packed basil leaves
I tablespoon olive oil
I clove garlic
2 tablespoons lemon juice
½ teaspoon salt

Instructions: Top and tail the courgettes. To make the linguine, slice them into thin strips using a mandoline or vegetable peeler. Stack strips on top of each other and slice them lengthways creating linguine strips. Combine all sauce ingredients in a high speed blender and place in a bowl with the courgette strips. Mix by hand to coat the linguine, leave for 5 minutes to allow flavour to infuse and serve.

....

Tip 10: As the size and water content of fresh ingredients vary, the recipes may differ slightly in quantity and consistency. Remember you can always add to a recipe but taking something out is a little harder so be sure to judge it, taste-testing and adding more seasoning or liquids as you go.

....

137

Lime and Ginger Stir Raw Marinade

Juice and zest of 1 lime
1 inch finely grated root ginger, peeled
1 clove garlic, pressed
2 tablespoons tamari
10 basil leaves, chiffonade (cut into long thin strips)
1 carrot, julienne
¼ cup red cabbage, thinly sliced
1 spring onion, finely chopped
¼ red pepper, thinly sliced
3 baby corn, thinly sliced

Instructions: Combine all ingredients in a bowl and leave to marinate for at least 15 minutes. Drain all ingredients and transfer to a plate discarding the remaining liquid.

....

Tip 11: Take advantage of online grocery shopping and set up your weekly basics when you're feeling well so you can get all you need delivered straight to your door on the days you're not feeling so great.

....

Pad Thai

1 carrot, julienned
1 courgette, thinly sliced using a vegetable peeler
1 spring onion, thinly sliced
1 red or yellow pepper, thinly sliced
1 small handful bean sprouts
1 small handful coriander, roughly chopped
5 basil leaves, chiffonade
2 tablespoons lime juice
1 tablespoon tamari

Instructions: Make linguine strips with the courgette as outlined in **Lemon Basil Linguine**. Combine all ingredients in a bowl and leave to marinate while making the Pad Thai sauce.

Pad Thai Sauce

2 tablespoons almond butter
2 tablespoons lime juice
1 teaspoon apple cider vinegar
2 tablespoons tamari
1 inch root ginger, peeled
1 clove garlic
1 teaspoon stevia
1 tablespoon water

Combine all sauce ingredients in a food processor until smooth but sticky. Drain the Pad Thai vegetables, and with your hands mix the Pad Thai Sauce in with the vegetables and serve.

Yellow Pepper Soup

1 cup carrot juice
½ cup carrot, chopped
2 sticks celery
1 avocado
4 medium-sized tomatoes
1 small handful coriander
1 inch ginger root, peeled
1 teaspoon salt
1 yellow pepper
½ cup water

Instructions: Juice approximately 4 carrots to make 1 cup of carrot juice. Place the carrot juice in a high-speed blender with all the ingredients except the avocado and blend until smooth. Finally, add in the avocado and process to incorporate. Warm the soup gently in a saucepan until finger-warm.

Watercress Soup

1 cup water
1 clove garlic
2 cups watercress
½ teaspoon salt
1 small handful coriander
1 tablespoon lime juice
1 avocado

Instructions: Place all of the ingredients in a blender except the avocado and process until smooth. Add in the avocado and blend to incorporate. Warm the soup gently in a saucepan until finger-warm.

....

Tip 12: By making soup in a blender and warming it very gently, the enzyme and nutrient content are maintained, optimizing the nutritional value.

....

Kale and Sesame salad

2-3 cups kale, de-stemmed
1 tablespoon cold-pressed sesame oil
2 tablespoons lemon juice
½ teaspoon salt
¼ tablespoon tahini
4 baby tomatoes
Pinch cayenne pepper
1 teaspoon agave nectar
1 tablespoon sesame seeds

Instructions: Strip the kale from its tough centre stem and combine in a bowl with the oil, salt and lemon juice. Massage with your hands until the kale begins to wilt. Add in the tahini, cayenne pepper and agave nectar mixing them in by hand. Add the tomatoes, sprinkle over the sesame seeds and serve immediately.

Pop-eye Hemp Salad

1 ½ cups tightly packed spinach leaves
6 baby tomatoes, halved
1 tablespoon sunflower seeds
2 tablespoons shelled hemp seeds
1 avocado, sliced
1 spring onion, sliced
1 teaspoon hemp protein powder

Instructions: Place the spinach in a bowl with the tomatoes, avocado and spring onion. Sprinkle over the sunflower seeds, hemp seeds and hemp protein powder. Serve with **Olive Oyl Dressing.** (See Dressings and Dips)

Sprout Salad

I large handful alfalfa and broccoli sprouts
I carrot, grated
I spring onion, sliced
¼ cucumber, diced

Instructions: Place all ingredients in a bowl and drizzle with **Orange Pecan Dressing** (see Dressings and Dips).

Dressings And Dips

Olive Oyl

2 tablespoons olive oil
1 tablespoon lemon juice
2 teaspoons apple cider vinegar
1 garlic clove, pressed
½ teaspoon salt

Instructions: Mix all ingredients together in a blender.

Green Sleaves

2 tablespoons hemp oil
1 tablespoon apple cider vinegar
1 tablespoon lemon juice
1 tablespoon fresh parsley
½ teaspoon salt

Instructions: Mix all ingredients together in a blender.

Turmeric Tornado

2 tablespoons olive oil
1 tablespoon apple cider vinegar
1 tablespoon lemon juice
1 garlic clove, pressed
¼ teaspoon turmeric
Pinch black pepper
½ teaspoon salt

Instructions: Mix all ingredients together in a blender.

Orange Pecan Dressing

1 tablespoon Pecan nut butter
3 tablespoons orange juice
2 sun-dried tomatoes (soaked for at least one hour to soften)
Sun-dried tomato soak water if required

Instructions: Mix all ingredients together in a blender. Add a drop of sun-dried tomato soak water if needed to help the mixture combine.

Top 5 Worst Offender Foods To Eliminate and Why

- Fizzy drinks: contain excessive amounts of sugar which may be cancer-causing.

- Coffee: highly addictive, acidic and stressful to the body.

- Meat: highly acidic, pro-inflammatory and contains IGF-1 which makes cancer grow.

- Cheese: contains pesticide and hormone residues, is pro-inflammatory and contains IGF-1 which makes cancer grow.

- Oils: Corn, canola, sunflower, soybean oil are all pro-inflammatory and contain excessive amounts of omega-6.

The Cancer Journey

Desserts

Juicy Lucy

Oranges

Instructions: Juice 3 oranges and freeze in ice lolly moulds – the number of lollies made will depend on the size of the oranges.

Ice lollies are great for those days when the treatment has left you with a **dry mouth** and drinking water and juice just isn't cutting it. Of course you can buy all sorts of ready-made ice-lollies but making your own is much more fun, inexpensive and healthier for you. Feel free to add apple, pear, strawberries or grapes to make different flavours – the possibilities are endless!

Banana Ice Cream

6 bananas

Instructions: Peel and slice the bananas, put them in a container or freezer bag and place in the freezer for at least 3 hours. Take the bananas out of the freezer, let them defrost for 5 minutes and blend in the food processor until creamy. You could add a cup of frozen raspberries to make raspberry ripple ice cream, top with nuts or drizzle with **Caramel Sauce.**

Caramel Sauce
½ cup almond milk (see page 132)
³/₄ cup coconut butter, warmed to liquefy
1 teaspoon vanilla extract
½ cup dates

Instructions: Combine all ingredients in a high-speed blender until smooth.

Berry Blue Pie

Base

1 cup walnuts
½ cup almond pulp (what is left over after making Almond Milk, see page 132)
½ teaspoon salt
2 tablespoons agave nectar
2 tablespoons coconut oil

Instructions: For the base, process the walnuts until finely ground. Add the remaining ingredients and process until the mixture starts to stick together. Transfer to a loose-bottomed 8 inch tin and press down firmly until level. Place in the fridge or freezer while making the filling.

Filling

2 cups cashews
⅓ cup agave nectar
2 cups blueberries
¼ cup coconut oil, warmed to liquefy

Decoration

1 cup blueberries

Instructions: Place all the filling ingredients except the coconut oil in a high-speed blender and process until smooth. (You may benefit from pre-soaking the cashew nuts for 1 hour if your machine isn't up to the challenge. Drain before using.) Add the oil and blend to incorporate. Remove the base from the fridge or freezer and pour over the filling. Smooth over the top and decorate with the remaining blueberries. Place in the freezer for 2 hours to set. Remove the pie from the loose-bottomed tin by slowly pushing the bottom of the tin up until it is free of the round part of the tin.

Frazzle Block

Have you ever wondered how a microwave works? Well in 1989, Swiss biologist and scientist Dr Hans Hertel studied the effects of microwaved food. He discovered that over time, significant changes in blood chemistry occurred after eating microwaved food. Red blood cell activity decreased, as did the body's good cholesterol, resulting in a weakened immune system and an increase in leukocyte levels, indicating toxicity and cell damage. Hopefully you'll think twice about nuking your next meal to smithereens!

Hydration – Are You Getting Enough?

We may be stating the obvious but staying hydrated is so important and very often overlooked on a daily basis. If you wait until you are thirsty to drink water, then you are considered to be very dehydrated. Some of the symptoms of dehydration are dry mouth, dry skin and dry eyes. Other signs of dehydration you may not recognise as dehydration include inflammation, constipation, fluid retention, low energy and immune dysfunction. When you consider that the brain consists of 76% water, muscle contains 75% and bone has 25%, it is clear that the body needs hydrating to work efficiently. On rising, we would recommend drinking a pint of water to help your body flush out any toxins which have accumulated over night. It has been fasting for 8 hours while you've been sleeping so, by sipping on a caffeine-filled cup of tea or coffee first thing, you are sending your body into a state of stress! If you want something hot, drink hot water with a squeeze of lemon. Although lemons are acidic, they become alkaline as soon as they are ingested, helping to cleanse the body and kick-start the metabolism. To re-hydrate you must simply drink more water and cut out diuretic drinks such as coffee, tea, fizzy drinks and alcohol as these dehydrate your body. Beware that most fizzy drinks contain aspartame which is carcinogenic – something you should avoid like the plague if diagnosed with cancer.

We would suggest you invest in a water filter or buy the cleanest spring water you can find as it has been scientifically proven that tap water contains hormones, toxic metals and pesticides which are harmful and give our body yet more toxicity to deal with. Our poor little livers!

CHAPTER 12

Potions and Lotions

Skincare And Household Products

Not only can we take control of what we put into our bodies, we must also be conscious of what we put *onto* it, as well as the environments we surround ourselves with. The skin is the biggest organ we have, and when we clog it up with creams and potions, that are made with the same chemicals found in some of the cleaning products under our kitchen sink, we really aren't doing ourselves any favours. "We're not joking."

Our everyday bathroom basics contain a host of harmful chemicals which add to the toxic soup our body has to contend with. Here are just a few of the worst offenders, to show you just how dangerous slathering on your favourite moisturiser can be.

Artificial colours and fragrances: some artificial colours have been linked to hyperactivity and attention deficit disorder (ADHD) and are a common cause of skin irritations and allergic reactions. They can be found in perfumes, scented products and cosmetics.

Formaldehyde: a toxic colourless gas which, when combined with water, is used as a preservative or disinfectant. It can trigger breathing difficulties such as asthma, and irritate the eyes, nose and throat. It is found in shampoos, deodorants, hand wash and other toiletries. It is a carcinogen (cancer-causing).

Phthalates: also known as 'gender benders' owing to their hormone-disrupting properties. They've been linked to deformed male reproductive organs in foetuses, and to decreased fertility in women. Found in lipstick, hairspray and nail polish.

Parabens: another 'gender bender' preservative used in cosmetics and toiletries.

Sodium Laurel Sulphate (SLS): a caustic cleanser that can cause irritation to the scalp, eyes and skin. It is found in shampoos, shower gels, toothpastes and even products 'suitable' for babies.

Obviously washing your hair once with carcinogenic shampoo isn't going to give you cancer. But it's the sheer volume of toxins that you may, unknowingly, be absorbing day in day out, that will cause the problems. Over time, these toxins stockpile, the body becomes overworked and with no way of being able to eliminate all of them, your body is unable to fight them and illness sets in. Coupled with a poor diet, a weakened immune system and stress, you'll be drowning in a sea of toxicity.

Although chemical free products are more expensive, it is definitely worth it. **You** are definitely worth it! Janey Lee-Grace, author of *Look Great Naturally...Without Ditching the Lipstick* offers great advice on how to go toxin-free inexpensively.

Check the Resources Section for online sources of chemical free products and information to help you transition to using cleaner, less toxic products.

All in all, by arming yourself with the knowledge of how to support your body by eating healthier foods, reducing stress and eliminating toxins you give yourself the best possible chance of overcoming illness, and living a life of health and happiness, cancer or no cancer.

Conclusion – Heaven Can Wait!

We know only too well that being diagnosed with cancer has a profound impact on our psychological wellbeing as well as our physical health. It's likely that you feel like Alice falling down a big black hole, with no magic potion to make it all better nor a key to open the door to a whole other world. We also know that if someone you love is diagnosed with cancer you may feel desperate and completely helpless. But please be assured that it doesn't have to be so. From our experience we know that family and friends can play a huge role in helping us deal with our situation – your support is incredibly important. Our hope is that this book will help anyone affected by a diagnosis of cancer to navigate the cancer journey.

The fact is, there is no map to cancer. What works for one person doesn't necessarily work for another, but there are some fundamental things that we have found to be useful and we hope our combined experiences will be of benefit to you. We've tried to give you lots of tips, a dash of inspiration and a bucket load of compassion to help you not only come to terms with your diagnosis but encourage you to reassess your priorities and give your life a new sense of purpose and meaning.

We know this journey can be scary, especially because no-one else can walk in your shoes except you. Take comfort from the fact that although you might feel like it, you're not alone. There are thousands, if not millions of people in a similar predicament to you and while no case is the same, someone will be able to relate to you and your story in some way. The support is there – please help yourself to it.

From dealing with your diagnosis, talking with your consultants, getting treatment, breaking the news to your friends and loved ones, we hope this book will help you navigate your journey. We hope you will choose to dip in and out of it, whether it be for dealing with your emotional needs, pampering your body and soul, understanding how you can choose what to eat to increase your odds for recovery or for great tips and recipes.

We really would recommend you try to find out as much as you can using the books and references we have provided, as we believe this will help you paint a clearer picture of how to get your body back to health. The purpose of this book is to enable you to empower yourself to take back the reins and regain some control. Remember it is your body, you do have choices in your treatment and there are lots of positive steps you can take to help yourself heal.

From the bottom of our hearts we wish you health and happiness. You are all in our thoughts.

Polly, Pam and Nick.

The Cancer Journey

Glossary

Acupuncture – This is the procedure of inserting and manipulating needles into various points on the body to aid relaxation. It is also thought to have therapeutic benefits such as relieving nausea and pain.

ADHD – Attention Deficit Hyperactivity Disorder is a developmental behavioural disorder which is characterised by problems with poor attention span and hyperactivity.

Angiogenesis – The process in which cancer cells send messages to nearby blood vessels causing new blood vessels to grow towards them. Theyn then hi-jack the blood supply for its own use which eventually resulting in a tumour.

Antiemetic – A drug that is used to prevent sickness and nausea.

Anti-Inflammatory – Refers to the property of a substance or treatment that reduces inflammation.

Antioxidant – A molecule capable of inhibiting the oxidation of other molecules such as free radicals which can start chain reactions that damage cells and lead to chronic disease.

Apoptosis – When the cancer cell decides to end its own life.

Aromatherapy – This is a form of complementary therapy that uses smell from aromatic oils to alter an individual's mood and effect calm and relaxation.

Aspartame – An artificial sweetener used as a sugar substitute.

Betacarotene – This is a naturally occurring organic compound and is responsible for the orange colour of many fruits and vegetables. It is converted to vitamin A in the body and has anti-oxidant properties.

Bromelain – Is a plant extract found in the juice and stems of pineapples. It is has natural anti-inflammatory properties.

Carcinogen/Carcinogenic – Any substance that is responsible for causing cancer.

Catechin – A type of antioxidant shown to inhibit the growth of cancer cells.

Cognitive Behaviour Therapy – A problem-solving type of psychotherapy designed to help people overcome their difficulties through changing their thinking, behaviour, and emotional response.

Diuretic – Diruetics are medicines that remove water from the body by increasing urine excretion.

EGCG (Epigallocatechin gallate) – A type of catechin.

Endorphins – Small protein molecules found in the nervous system which are naturally released by the body in response to stress or pain. As well as blocking pain signals they can also produce feelings of euphoria (the 'runners high' is a good example of this).

Enzymes – These are proteins that catalyse biological reactions.

Flavenoids – Have anti-oxidant properties which are thought to kill cancer cells and prevent/inhibit tumour invasion.

Free radical – An atom or group of atoms that are unstable and possess an odd number of electrons. Free radicals can cause DNA damage and contribute to illness and disease.

Glycaemic Index (GI) – This is a numerical scale used to indicate the effects of food on blood glucose (blood sugar) level.

Lentinan – This is a compound derived from shiitake mushrooms and is a type of polysaccharide which can increase tumour death.

Leukocyte – These are white blood cells and are cells of the immune system.

Leukocytosis – When the white blood cell count is raised above the normal range in the blood and usually happens in response to infection.

Limbic system – This is the part of the brain which controls emotions.

Lycopene – Lycopene is a phytochemical and is part of the carotenoid family. It has anti-oxidant properties and is thought to be beneficial in both prevention and treatment of some types of cancer.

Lymph fluid – This is a fluid which occupies the space between cells and is similar to blood plasma. It contains white blood cells and the lymph picks up foreign cells, bacteria and debris and transfers them to lymph nodes where they are destroyed.

Lymphoedema – A condition of localized fluid retention and tissue swelling caused by a compromised or sluggish lymphatic system.

Meditation – This is a technique where one can learn to train the brain to cultivate a feeling of internal calm and a positive state of mind.

Metastasis – The spread of a disease from one organ or part of the body to another.

Methylsulfonylmethane (MSM) – A naturally occurring compound which is used as a nutritional supplement. It is considered to be helpful in reducing pain and inflammation.

Neural Pathways – Connect one part of the nervous system with another. They consist of bundles of neurons (nerves) and dictate how messages and information are passed around the nervous system.

Pathogens – An infectious germ that causes disease to its host.

PCBs – Polychlorinated biphenyls. These are a group of man-made compounds which were widely used in the past, mainly in electrical equipment. Due to their toxicity, harmful effects on health and classification as an environmental pollutant they were banned, but because they are generally very stable they are still found in the environment.

Phytonutrient – The term used to describe plant compounds which are thought to have health-protecting qualities.

Phytochemical – A chemical compound that occurs naturally in plants and is a term generally used to refer to those chemicals that may positively affect health.

Polysaccharides – Are carbohydrates such as starch and cellulose.

Polyphenol – A chemical compound believed to have antioxidant characteristics and thought to reduce the risk of cardiovascular disease and cancer.

Probiotics – Live microorganisms (in most cases, bacteria) that are beneficial to the health and balance of the human gut. They are also called 'friendly' or 'good' bacteria.

Reiki – This a system of natural healing which evolved in Japan and is useful for stress reduction, relaxation and is also believed to promote healing.

Reflexology – Reflexology is the practice of applying pressure to the feet and hands and has been demonstrated to promote relaxation and to help relieve cancer pain and also some symptoms and side effects associated with cancer treatment.

QiGong – A Chinese form of Martial Arts, Qigong practice involves the manipulation and balance of the qi (energy) within the practitioner's body and its interaction with the practitioner's surroundings.

Resveratrol – A substance found in red grapes thought to have anti-inflammatory and anti-cancer properties.

Visualisation -Is the technique of using one's imagination to create an image of a specific outcome occurring and this can subsequently have a positive effect on your mind and body.

Resources

Websites
Diet and Lifestyle Information and Inspiration
www.pollynoble.com
www.crazysexylife.com
www.drmercola.com
www.credence.org
www.shazzie.com
www.katesmagicbubble.com
www.healthcreation.co.uk
www.imperfectlynatural.com
www.puremamas.squarespace.com
www.thekindlife.com
www.davidwolfe.com

Coaching
www.willtolivecoaching.com
www.pollynoble.com
www.thebig-leap.com

Raw food Information and Recipes
www.pollynoble.com
www.therawchef.com
www.aniphyo.com
www.kristensraw.com
www.betterraw.com
www.kefir.net

Raw Food Delivery and Box Scheme Information
www.rawfairies.com
www.riverford.co.uk
www.boxscheme.org
www.bigbarn.co.uk

Food and Superfood Stockists

www.detoxyourworld.com
www.rawliving.eu
www.lionheartherbs.com
www.gojiking.co.uk
www.naturallygreen.co.uk
www.fresh-network.com
www.tea4life.co.uk
www.godshaer.co.uk
www.e3live.com
www.naked-chocolate.com
www.chocchick.com

Supplements

www.udoschoice.co.uk
www.aggressivehealthshop.com
www.e3live.com

Wheatgrass delivery and Sprouting

www.wheatgrass-uk.com

Juice Extractors

www.juicemaster.com
www.eujuicers.com/en
www.ukjuicers.com
www.juiceland.com

Water

www.danielvitalis.com
www.deesidewater.co.uk

Raw Food Restaurants

www.safrestaurant.com
www.vitaorganic.co.uk
www.inspiralled.net
www.vantra.co.uk

Chemical-Free Products

www.lovelula.com
www.lavera.co.uk
www.greenpeople.co.uk
www.nealsyardremedies.com
www.jowoodorganics.com
www.coconoil.com
www.drhaushka.co.uk
www.iamnatural.co.uk
www.cosmeticdatabase.com

Meditation and Mind Body Healing

www.sandynewbigging.com
www.livingmagically.co.uk
www.drdavidhamilton.com
www.mind-springs.org
www.stillnessbuddy.com

Cancer Support

The Cancer Journey – www.thecancerjourneybook.com
Yes To Life – www.yestolife.org.uk
CANCERactive – www.canceractive.com
Wallace Cancer Care – www.wallacecancercare.org.uk
Teenage Cancer Trust – www.teenagecancertrust.org
Macmillan – www.macmillan.org.uk
Marie Curie – www.mariecurie.org.uk
Never Alone – www.neveralone.org
Penny Brohn Cancer Care – www.pennybrohncancercare.org

Detox Centres

Hippocrates Health Institute – www.hippocratesinst.org
Ann Wigmore Natural Health Institute – www.annwigmore.org
Gerson Institute – www.gerson.org
Detox International – www.detox-international.com

Other Useful Websites
www.thework.com by Byron Katie
www.ewg.org – Environmental Working Group
www.wen.org.uk – Women's Environmental Network

Books

Diet and Lifestyle
Anti-Cancer – A New Way of Life by Dr David Servan Schreiber.
Penguin Books, ISBN 978-0-718-15929-5

C: Because Cowards Get Cancer Too by John Diamond.
Vermillion, London. ISBN 978-0091816650

Living Food for Health by Gillian McKeith, Piatkus Books, ISBN 978-0749925406

Crazy Sexy Diet by Kris Carr, Skirt! ISBN 978-1599218014

The Body Ecology Diet: Recovering Your Health and Rebuilding Your Immunity by Donna Gates and Linda Schatz, Hay House ISBN 978-1401935436

The New Glucose Revolution: Low GI Eating Made Easy by Jennie Brand – Miller, MD, Kaye- Foster Powell and Philippa Sandall, Marlowe & Co, ISBN 978-1569243855

The Rainbow Diet and How It Can Help You Beat Cancer by Chris Woollams, Health Issues Ltd, ISBN 978-0954296896

The China Study: The Most Comprehensive Study of Nutrition Ever Conducted – Startling Implications for Diet, Weight Loss and Long-term Health by T. Colin Campbell, BenBella Books, ISBN 978-1932100662

The Sprouters Handbook by Edward Cairney, Argyll Publishing, ISBN 978-1874640486

Sprout Garden by Mark Matthew Braunstein, Book Publishing Company, ISBN 978-1570670732

Detoxify or Die by Sherry A. Rogers,MD, Prestige Pubs,ISBN 978-1887202046

The Acid-Alkaline Diet for Optimum Health by Christopher Vasey and Jon Graham, Healing Arts Press, **ISBN 0892810998**

Look Great Naturally Without Ditching the Lipstick by Janey Lee Grace, Hay House UK, ISBN 978-1848502031

Pure Living by Sally Bevan (How to transform your home into a haven) BBC Publications, ISBN 978-0563488798

Raw Food
Green For Life by Victoria Boutenko
Atlantic Books, ISBN 978-1556439308

Living Raw Food by Sarma Melngailis, William Morrow Cookbooks, ISBN 978-0061458477

Living on Live Food by Alissa Cohen, Cohen Publishing, ISBN 0-9748963-0-6

Ani's Raw Food Essentials by Ani Phyo, Da Capo ISBN 978-0738213774

Going Raw: Everything You Need to Start Your Own Raw Food Diet & Lifestyle Revolution at Home by Judita Wignall, Quarry Books, ISBN 978-1592536856

Cooked Food

Go Dairy Free: The Guide and Cookbook for Milk Allergies, Lactose Intolerance, and Casein-free Living by Alisa Marie Fleming, Fleming Ink, ISBN 978-0979128622

The Kind Diet: A Simple Guide to Feeling Great, Losing Weight, and Saving the Planet by Alicia Silverstone, Rodale Incorporated, ISBN 978-1609611354

Juicing

The Juice Masters Ultimate Fast Food by Jason Vale, Thorsons, ISBN 978-0007156795

The Big Book of Juices by Natalie Savona, Duncan Baird Publishers, ISBN 978-1904292234

The Wheatgrass Book by Ann Wigmore, Avery Publishing Book, ISBN 978-0895292346

Healing, Creativity and Self-Expression

How Your Mind Can Heal Your Body by Dr David Hamilton. Hay House, ISBN 978-1848500235

On Death and Dying by Elizabeth Kübler-Ross. Routledge, ISBN 0415040159

Peace is Every Step by Thich Nhat Hanh. Bantam Books, ISBN 0-553-35139-7

Opening Up – The Healing Power of Expressing Emotions by Dr James W Pennebaker, The Guildford Press, ISBN 1-57230-238-0 Mindfulness Meditation for Everyday Life by Jon Kabat-Zinn. Piatkus, ISBN 0-7499-1422

The Artist's Way by Julia Cameron, Pan Books, ISBN 978-033034358-9

Loving What Is by Byron Katie, Rider Books, ISBN 9780712629300

Everything You Need To Know to Help You Beat Cancer by Chris Woollams, Health Issues Ltd, ISBN 0-9542968-5-0

Conscious Medicine by Gill Edwards, Piatkus, ISBN 978-0749941987

Communication skills
How to make people like you in 90 seconds or less by Nichols Boothman, Workman Publishing, ISBN 978-0761149460

59 Seconds by Richard Wiseman, Macmillan, ISBN 978-0-230-74429-5

Influence – The Psychology of Persuasion by Robert B. Cialdini PhD, Collins, ISBN 978-0-06-124189-5

Straw Dogs by Professor John Gray, Granta Books London, ISBN978-1-86207-596-2

References

Walker, L.G., Walker, M.B., Simpson, F., et al (1997). Guided imagery and relaxation therapy can modify host defences in women receiving treatment for locally advanced breast cancer. British Journal of Surgery 84 (15 Suppl 1): 31.

Dixon, 1998. Does 'healing' benefit patients with chronic symptoms? A quasi-randomized trial in general practice. Journal of the Royal Society of Medicine 91: 183-189.

Luebbert, K., Dahme, B. & Hasenbring, M. (2001). The effectiveness of relaxation training in reducing treatment-related symptoms and improving emotional adjustment in acute non-surgical cancer treatment: a meta-analytical review. Psycho-oncology, 10 (6): 490-502.

Kolcaba, K. & Fox, C. (1999). The effects of guided imagery on comfort of women with early stage breast cancer undergoing radiation therapy. Oncology Nursing Forum. 26(1): 67-72.

Roffe, L., Schmidt, K. & Ernst, E. (2005). A systematic review of guided imagery as an adjuvant cancer therapy. Psycho-Oncology. 14(8): 607-617.

Walker, L.G., Walker, M.B., Ogston, K., Heys, S.D., Ah-See, A.K., Miller, I.D., Hutcheon, A.W., Sarkar, T.K. & Eremin, O. (1999). Psychological, clinical and pathological effects of relaxation training and guided imagery during primary chemotherapy. British Journal of Cancer. 80(1-2): 262-268.

Koppikar, S.J., Choudhari, A.S., Suryavabshi, S.A., Kumari, S., Chattopadhyay, S. and Kaul-Ghanekar, R., (2010) Aqueous cinnamon extract (ACE-c) from the bark of Cinnamomum cassia causes apoptosis in human cervical cancer cell line (SiHa) through loss of mitochondrial membrane potential. BMC Cancer 10:210

Kwon, H.K., Hwang, J.S., So, J.S., Lee, C.G., Sahoo, A., Ryu, J.H., Jeon, W.K., Ko, B.S., Im, C.R., lee, C.R. Park, Z.Y. and Im, S.H. (2010). Cinnamon extract induces tumor cell death through inhibition of NFkappaB and API. BMC Cancer 10:392

Index

The Cancer Journey